FINDING SUTTON'S CHOICE
A Novel

By Brenda Haas

Praise for *Finding Sutton's Choice*

"A beautiful story about forgiveness, second chances, and finding home in unexpected places. If you've ever wrestled with family messes or avoided going back to the town that raised you, you'll enjoy this one. I'd recommend it to readers who enjoy emotionally driven fiction with depth, especially fans of Ann Patchett or Elizabeth Berg."
—Literary Titan

"Haas writes with skill and assurance, rendering the waterfront community in vivid detail and giving Charlotte's inner conflicts emotional depth without slowing the story's momentum. Her prose is grounded and filled with flashes of sardonic wit... The novel succeeds as a moving account of strained family bonds, illness, and second chances. A tender family story with familiar beats, elevated by strong characters and engaging prose."
—Kirkus Reviews

"A beautifully crafted story about love, loss, and family ties, set against the nostalgic backdrop of small-town America. Haas's storytelling is top-notch and skillfully relatable as she challenges readers to reflect on their relationships and the complexities that come with them. A must-read for anyone seeking a heartfelt narrative that will stay with them long after turning the last page."
—Susan Poole, author of *Out of the Crash*

"Surprising, deep, and—ultimately—a beautiful picture of family dynamics, coming-of-age, and the true meaning of love. Have tissues beside you."
—Laurel Houck, author of *Searching for Home*

"A book that absorbed my mind and my heart. An intelligently written, engaging novel filled with unique, charming characters. Those who live in or visit the real-life community of Lakeside, Ohio, will find the connections poignantly entertaining. Those who haven't visited Lakeside will want to after reading *Finding Sutton's Choice*."
—Sheri Trusty, Editor, *The Beacon*, a Lake Erie newspaper

"Going home has never felt more real. This heartfelt family drama makes us reflect on whether our perceptions about childhood tell our full story and also question whether there is room for understanding and forgiveness."
—Traci Richards, Owner, Millie Magoo's & The Fine Print bookstore

"A thoughtful exploration of memory, identity, and the fragile architecture of family. With a narrative that balances emotional resonance and thematic depth, Alzheimer's becomes more than a plot device—it becomes a lens through which generational disconnect is refracted. Haas writes with a deep appreciation for the cost of memory's erosion, capturing how grief, love, and the fog of forgetting intersect in daily life. *Finding Sutton's Choice* lingers in the spaces between memory and myth, asking what it means to truly know someone—especially when memory fails."
—RedReviews4You, Goodreads

"I couldn't put it down! We all make choices every day, and those choices have consequences. Ms. Haas has created a world peopled by real, imperfect, likable characters dealing with life's little surprises. I laughed and I cried right along with them. Ms. Haas deserves to be read!"
—Susan J. Holloway, Amazon

"A great read. Well written and touching story that is highly relatable to most of us (or will be). I especially appreciate the character development. Looking forward to the author's next work."
—Danny Moulton, Amazon

"I had the best time reading *Finding Sutton's Choice*... I thought this book really explored ideas of grief and loss of a parent very well."
—Lauren, Goodreads

"Brenda Haas has created a tale set in Lakeside, Ohio, and her wonderful descriptions of Lake Erie make it feel like one of the characters."
—Melissa J., Books 4 Days

"What a wonderful book! You laugh, you tear up, you cheer, and you reflect on your own childhood memories."
—Regina Bryant, Amazon

For Mike, because you knew I could.

And for the Johns, the Gwens, the Kens, and the Sues
of the world.
Your memories remain with those who will never forget you.

1

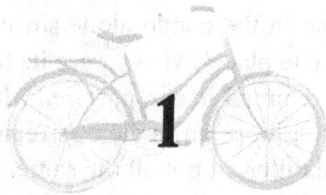

Charlotte Sutton glanced at the buzzing phone lying beside her on the window seat.

Area code 419. Lakeside, Ohio. Frowning, she set her laptop aside and silenced the call, placing her cell face-down.

It's nothing. A telemarketer.

Or was it? In recent weeks, she'd received more than one dropped call from her Lake Erie hometown—an unlikely occurrence on any day of any week of any month. A boy—a teenager—had left a message the night before. He'd stumbled through a request to discuss Chuck and hung up without giving his name.

Charlotte hadn't returned the call. If some star-struck, wannabe athlete required her esteemed father's advice, autograph, or approval, he was looking in the wrong dugout. He'd need to do a search of "Chuck Sutton," "retired baseball player," "author," "shitty dad," or some-such combination. She wasn't Chuck's publicist.

Shoving the ungracious thought back into her closet full of demons, Charlotte turned her attention to the old brownstone apartments across the street. A glint of rare November sunshine reflected off the metal fire escape snaking from a rooftop martini bar to the

Pittsburgh sidewalk below, where people in business attire scurried like an army of ants. In equal numbers, tourists and locals meandered from shop window to shop window. A homeless man squatted on a cardboard square on the stoop of an abandoned storefront. To her left, Charlotte glimpsed a small section of the Roberto Clemente Bridge, its straw-colored arch an icon of the city of black and gold. She could even see a corner of the baseball stadium. Ironic, really. She hated baseball—something her father would never understand.

Charlotte had lived in the condo alone since her mother remarried and moved on. The place's views were its biggest selling point, but the novelty had dimmed in the past year. It was like watching a cityscape video on a loop—an endless, streaming melting pot of faceless strangers, all different but all the same.

She drained the remains of her coffee, hurried across the room, and plunked the mug into the sink. The sailboat etched onto its side served as a niggling reminder of the call from the lake.

It's nothing. Absolutely nothing. Charlotte returned to the window and glanced at the bricks of the baseball stadium.

"Dammit." *It's probably something.* She snapped up her cell and retrieved the message.

"Hello," the caller said. "My name is Jake Forrester. I'm trying to get in touch with Charlie Sutton."

Charlie. The use of the familiar, masculine moniker sent a twitch up Charlotte's spine.

"We haven't met," Jake said. "I'm a friend of your father's. I understand you're quite busy, Charlie—"

"Aah, hell no." Charlotte dropped the message and threw the phone onto the cushions. This Jake person, who had no right whatsoever to use the wretched, awful nickname, sounded... crisp and business-like. Definitely *not* a teenager. He was a reporter. Had to be. She'd endured countless interviews when she was still under her father's roof. Chuck had always introduced her as his daughter "Charlie," as if Charlotte was a derivative of Charles. God, she hated the name. And nicknames, in general. They'd been as common as trailer parks and fishing poles when she was growing up. Scooter and Babs and Bubbles and Pop-Tart. Everybody had a nickname. Charlotte had been saddled with more than one.

It doesn't matter. Not anymore.

Charlotte tucked a short wisp of dark hair behind her ear. Dismissing her past, she returned to her laptop and carefully scanned the final draft of her essay about growing up an only child. Finding no errors, she pressed "send" to her editor. A faint smile edged her lips with the click of the button, and her gaze shifted to the opposite wall. The framed two-page spread of her first published magazine article hung there. Her miniature headshot stared back at her.

Charlotte's smile faded. Even from a distance, she recognized the acute resemblance to her father.

"This is bullshit." She grabbed her keys and the spare to the apartment down the hall, pulled the door shut behind her, and hurried to #517. Expecting no one home, she gave a light tap and shoved the key in the hole. A muffled *woof* greeted her from the other side. Charlotte entered, and a large blur of light fur bounded toward her.

"Good boy, Alfredo. How's my buddy?" She bent down to the Labrador retriever circling her legs. "You're just what I need right now. Elliot still at work, huh? Wanna go for a walk?"

She pulled a leash from a wall hook, ignoring the flicker of guilt that pushed her toward the door. There would be an awkward conversation. No avoiding it. Her ex would see this as a sign—a grand sign of reconciliation and invitation.

It was not a sign, and there would be nothing grand about it.

"Charlotte? What are you doing here?"

"Oh." Charlotte turned. Elliot stood in his bedroom doorway. Tall and lean, he wore pressed khakis paired with a red polo—a walking insurance commercial. His dark eyes showed not one ounce of concern that she was standing, uninvited, in his apartment.

"Hey," Charlotte mumbled.

"It's great to see you." Elliot strode across the room and enveloped her in a hug. "What's it been? Two weeks?"

"About." Charlotte backed up a step. "I didn't think you'd be home."

Elliot blinked.

Damn it. Charlotte's nails bit into her palms. It was never her goal to be rude; she just had a knack for saying the wrong thing. In the wrong way. Every. Single. Time.

She shook her head. "I'm sorry. I didn't mean it that way. I just... I should have called first. I needed a little pet therapy and thought maybe Alfredo would like to go for a walk. I know it's not my usual day to walk him. I thought you'd be at the office."

"I delivered a project for Tania on the south side then had a dentist appointment. See?" Elliot smiled, his polished teeth gleaming. "I'm taking the rest of the day off. Why don't we *all* take that walk? I have so much to tell you. We'll go down by the fountain to our usual spot." He took a breath, his gaze trained on hers. "If that's okay?"

So earnest and well-meaning, like Alfredo.

"Um, sure," Charlotte said.

Elliot grabbed his coat and some dog treats, and Charlotte shooed Alfredo into the hallway. The dog took the lead down five flights of stairs, and they exited onto the sidewalk. Despite Thanksgiving being weeks away, the city dripped with red and green decorations.

"So, are you still on the car dealership account?" Elliot said. "I haven't seen you in the office."

"Yeah." Charlotte frowned. "I've been doing a lot from home." Her part-time gig with Beyond Business, the Pittsburgh advertising agency where they both worked, brought her a step closer to being a full-time writer. Whether she'd gotten the job because of Elliot or, worse, because of her last name, she didn't like to consider too closely.

They meandered in a westerly direction, weaving through a sea of lunchtime city strollers. Elliot chattered beside Charlotte, talking about the meal he'd cooked the previous night and the plot of a rom-com he'd seen without her and how pleased he was with the shirt he'd bought the previous day. Charlotte barely registered his monologue. She couldn't stop thinking about the phone call.

It had been a decade since she left.

Not nearly long enough.

Any reminder of her father, and his Chuck ways, never failed to stir her up—a red-hot anger making her head hurt and her palms sweat. It should have been different, but she couldn't change the past.

His loss. Not mine. How can you lose something you never really had?

Charlotte paused near the park's fountain, her breath pluming white before her. Alfredo shoved his body against her knee.

Elliot lengthened his stride. "And when I took Alfredo to the groomer the other day, they gave me a—"

"I wonder what the hell he's up to now," Charlotte muttered.

Elliot turned. "Did you say something?"

"Nothing."

"Are you okay, Charlotte?"

"Sure. Fine."

A nearby couple swung a giggling toddler between their outstretched hands. The child yelled, "Again. Again." Charlotte's own father was a stranger; no amount of peeling back layers would make him less so. Why would someone call about him? Why should it have anything at all to do with her?

"Why did you need pet therapy? What happened?"

"Nothing. Got a call from home about my dad."

"Huh." Elliot's voice dropped. "Is everything okay?"

"I'm not sure, to be honest." Charlotte pulled the phone from her pocket. She held it, not really seeing it, allowing the screen to remain dark a bit longer. "Can you give me a second? I need to check something." She walked to the water's edge and pressed a button.

"Hello. My name is Jake Forrester. I'm trying to get in touch with Charlie Sutton. We haven't met. I'm a friend of your father's. I understand you're quite busy, Charlie, but Chuck hasn't been himself recently. We're worried about him. The doctors are still running some tests, but it would be best if you came home, if you can spare the time. Please, at least call. Your dad may have Alzheimer's."

"Oh." Charlotte dropped her cell, her numb fingers hovering in mid-air, forgotten.

* * * * *

Guilt and her usual sense of duty gnawed a hole in Charlotte's stomach during the entire three-hour drive from Pittsburgh the next day.

Waves lapped at the rocks on either side of the causeway spanning Sandusky Bay, offering a wet "hello" to an old friend. A motorboat darted from point A to point B with the precision of a surgeon's scalpel, quite the opposite of the meandering sailboat Charlotte had often guided across Lake Erie.

Bowing to tradition, she began counting the seagulls perched on top of the bridge's light poles. They stood like mini statues, their beaks facing into the wind. The sight lifted her spirits a bit, reminding her of rides in the back of her parents' sedan, back before the divorce. She'd tally the birdie sentinels every time the family crossed Sandusky Bay. In good weather, with every pole occupied, they'd totaled 50? 70? 100? But it was windy; only a fraction of those numbers welcomed Charlotte this day. She barely glanced at the sign for the Lakeside Marblehead exit and turned toward the peninsula.

"Let me know when you get in." Elliot's disembodied voice squawked from the car speaker. "You'll do that? Call me? Otherwise, I'll think you were in an accident. You won't get in an accident, will you?"

Charlotte sighed and adjusted the volume. She should never have taken Alfredo for that walk.

"I won't get in an accident. I'm almost there."

"I sure hope your dad is okay. I'm one of his biggest fans. I've told you that, right? Does he still play any ball? I mean, I bet he was something to watch out on the field when you were a kid. Must have been cool as hell. Did he coach your little league?"

"Chuck didn't coach shit. He was hardly around." Charlotte sounded whiny, and she hated herself for it.

"Oh."

"He left baseball, published his book... divorced my mother."

And forgot I existed.

In that order.

"Oh."

"Honestly? I barely know him."

He'd missed most of Charlotte's games. Softball. Basketball. Volleyball. Every sport she tried. Chuck's spot on the bleachers next to Mom had often remained a gaping hole between spectators. A constant distraction. An endless, pointless wondering if the vacancy might be filled between foul balls.

Stupid baseball.

"Huh. I wouldn't have expected that," Elliot said. "I'm sorry, Charlotte."

"Yeah. Me, too," Charlotte said. "I'm sorry about a lot of things."

"We dated for nearly six months. How come you never told me much about when you were growing up?"

"I don't like to relive it."

"I see." Elliot paused. "So, does the lake freeze? I suppose not in November. Are there boats on the water? Send me pictures."

"Sure."

"You need me to let Tania know you're gone? I can do that. No problem. Really. I'll—"

Charlotte sighed. "Relax, Elliot. I've already told her. She'll email me if she needs something."

"You're coming home Monday, right? What time? Before dinner? I'll make fettuccine—your favorite."

"That's Alfredo's favorite."

"Oh, gosh." Elliot laughed. "You're right. Well, I'll make you something. How about lasagna?"

Charlotte's fingers gripped the steering wheel. "Sorry. I don't think I'll be home by dinner. Gotta go. Bad reception."

"Oh. Well, good luck with your dad. I'm here if you need me."

"I know. And... thanks, Elliot." Swallowing air and an urge to cry, Charlotte dropped the call. He was suffocating her with love and lasagna.

Their relationship, or whatever one wished to call it, had been on-again, off-again more times than she cared to count. Elliot meant well, but he deserved someone in a better mental space than she was or probably ever would be. She just couldn't deal with it. Not on top of the whole Chuck thing.

They were off-again, and she intended to keep it that way.

Exiting, she passed a string of marine stores, many closed for the off-season. Bergman's roadside farmstand featured Halloween pumpkins and colorful mums. She debated stopping for her favorite peach preserves but continued on, absorbing the changes that had occurred over the years, but unphased by how much had remained the same.

Trailer park. Trailer park. Marina.

Marina. Marina. Trailer park.

Charlotte loosened her grip on the steering wheel and wiped one sweaty palm on her jeans and then the other. She slowed behind a rusty pick-up pulling a sleek, red motorboat. What would the weekend hold? For sure, Chuck would be surprised. They had not spoken since her and her mother's move to Pittsburgh right after high school graduation—one of many milestones Chuck had missed. That he hadn't left a message himself, instead of having the Jake person do it, pissed her off. Not that she was any better. Even a short return to Lakeside could... probably *would*... prove to be a bad idea. She hadn't called the Jake person back. She'd rather show up unannounced in case she changed her mind.

She passed Runinmuck campgrounds, and the car rolled to a stop at a food market on the corner. Ahead, Lakeside's entrance sign, in the shape of a gabled cottage roof, spanned the width of the road. Metal fences, like braces on invisible teeth, branched out from either side, providing a clear barrier to the one-square-mile resort community. Two unmanned ticket booths bided time until another busy summer season brought the gates down.

Charlotte had ventured beyond Lakeside's borders after graduation, searching for something less binding.

Something bigger. *Better.*

Yet here she was. Back again.

"I must be out of my damned mind." Charlotte inched her foot off the brake and allowed the vehicle to slowly creep through the booths and onto Lakeside property.

2

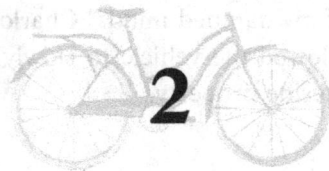

Named for a number (east and west) or a tree (north and south), the narrow streets featured a dense jumble of cottages on both sides. Most sported their own, personal nickname—Makin' Waves, Branch Office, The Old Salt, Lily's Pad—which Charlotte should have found annoying, not nostalgic. Some cottages, with garishly painted shaker-style siding, reminded her of the miniature dollhouse she'd spent hours playing with as a child, making up family stories in which only she knew the ending.

Lakeside provided a step back in time—like being dropped onto an old-timey movie set instead of landing in a genuine, 1800s Victorian village, sassed up and given hot running water to satisfy the modern-day visitor. Memories of sailing, shuffleboard tournaments, and fishing off the dock filtered through her mind like a slide deck. She tapped a nervous rhythm on the steering wheel and rolled her head. The tension along her shoulders tightened further.

It hasn't changed, even if I have.

Charlotte turned onto Pine. On her left, a shadow loomed and wavered on a screened porch. She frowned. She had missed Lake Erie and her many personalities—bathwater calm, wild waves, ice sculptures forming over the rocky shore. But she sure as hell had *not* missed living in a small town where everybody knew everybody's business—her family's, in particular.

It hadn't helped that Chuck Sutton was practically a local celebrity, and he collected friends like baseball cards. Her mother had called him "Good-time Charlie" for a reason. Where there was Chuck, there was always a party.

Charlotte preferred the anonymity of city life—blending in, being left alone, no longer a source of gossip. Her Pittsburgh neighbors were strangers. She liked it that way. She'd gained virtually no followers in her 28 years, except maybe Elliot.

And she was absolutely okay with being the opposite of a good time.

Proud of it, even.

The town's rumor chain, shorter in the off-season but still ferociously efficient, would barely give her time to park the car before everyone knew she was back. Wouldn't matter. She wasn't sticking around for long.

Charlotte crept onto the street, dead-ending into the waterfront. A sliver of Lake Erie appeared in the distance, and her heartbeat quickened. As if drawn there of its own volition, the car veered toward a pale-peach waterfront cottage with white scalloped trim that swooped and swirled from every edge of the pointed roof like frosting on a gingerbread house. Charlotte pulled into the lot between the cottage and the neighboring Hotel Lakeside, a three-story, lady-like behemoth with a screened-in front porch. An older model SUV, likely Chuck's, was the only vehicle parked there.

Killing the engine, Charlotte gazed up at the rear of the cottage. Her father had lived alone there since she and her mother left. A wooden sign in the shape of a sailboat listed above the back door, its hand-painted letters—a product of Charlotte's preteen creativity—faded but still legible.

Sutton's Choice.

Her father could have afforded to renovate it any way he wanted, but the cottage, in the family for more than six generations, had not changed much. Even the Rusty Banana—Charlotte's yellow tank-of-a-bike—still guarded the back door. Its chains were slick with oil, and the basket on the front looked new.

Odd. Chuck had always preferred to get his exercise strolling the perimeter of the community. Charlotte crept from her car and almost toppled a baseball bat propped against the porch step.

Is he living in the past?

Approaching the back door, she knocked and waited.

Knocked again.

Nothing.

Nerves resisting the movement, she grasped the knob. The door was unlocked, like always, and she poked her head inside the dimly lit kitchen.

"Anybody home? Chuck?"

A silence blanketed the place, like it was waiting for someone.

Questions buzzed in her head, but Charlotte refused to cross over the threshold uninvited. She yanked the door shut, hurried to the front of the house, and stopped.

The winds swirled leaves across the lawn fronting Lake Erie, and spray arched onto the wide swath of grass dominated by twin Cottonwood trees, their side-by-side trunks each at least three feet in diameter.

But it was the lake that drew Charlotte's attention.

The surface roiled, shimmering blue, silver, and gray. Whitecaps crested in the distance, sweeping in continuous waves toward the rock retaining wall along the water's edge.

Whoa. Chuck would say the ol' girl is angry.

And exactly what Charlotte needed. Despite its turbulent temperament, the large body of water provided a balm—a calming presence to be counted on. They understood each other—the lake and Charlotte Sutton.

I've missed you, my friend.

Charlotte took a deep, cleansing breath. It would be okay. It had to be.

Her gaze followed the footpath snaking along the shoreline. To the right of Sutton's Choice sprawled the hotel and a two-story pavilion with a long dock jutting out into the water. Regardless of what happened—how quickly she got back in her car and escaped—she would take a walk to the end of the dock.

She must. It was a time-honored Lakeside tradition—an itch that must be scratched.

First, she must locate Chuck. Charlotte turned west. Being a Saturday, she supposed she'd find her father at Shores Marina, either working or drinking.

Located just a block away and beyond the Lakeside fence, the marina looked out of place next to its genteel neighbors. A neon sign, gaudy and inconsistently blinking, announced The Surly Sturgeon, an attached sports bar and restaurant beside the bait shop fronting the docks. A dance hall in the 1800s, the squat building's puce-colored paint peeled in strips from the cement block beneath. Her father's office was housed in the rear, though Charlotte had never been in it. The rental income from his newspaper, and the fishing and drinking habits of the locals, kept Shores Marina afloat.

Charlotte approached an unlocked gate along the fence. She skirted The Surly Sturgeon and stopped at a door at the back of the building.

"You lookin' for someone in par-ti-cu-lar, honey? Huh? Shit-fire, it's colder than a witch's ass out here."

Charlotte turned. Beatrice Douglas, the marina owner, stood in the bar's main entrance. No taller than Charlotte's armpit, the sixty-something wore work boots, jeans rolled to a cuff, and an orange and brown flannel shirt. Her baseball cap—heralding the "#1 Surly Sturgeon"—topped a gray buzz cut.

"Hey, Ms. Douglas," Charlotte said. "Um, I was just looking for—"

"Charlie Sutton? Lordy, girl." The block of a woman lunged, threw her arms around Charlotte's middle, and pressed her face into Charlotte's chest. "Crap on a cracker." She tilted her head back and squinted. "You're all growed up."

"Yeah, Ms. Douglas. Um—"

"Call me Bea, dear. You're not 12 anymore, for devil's sake."

"Oh. Well, um—"

"Spit it out, girly. Quit your ummin' and into the bar with ya'." Bea grabbed Charlotte by the elbow and practically chucked her through the door. The room was dark, a bit musty-smelling, and quite deserted.

"You're gonna' need warmer clothes up here, or you'll catch your death by Thanksgiving. Been a cold, windy fall so far, and they say winter'll be a bitch. Truth be told, them Nor'easters can damn near freeze a wet fart. Take a seat."

Charlotte inched down onto a barstool. Only one of The Surly Sturgeon's big-screen televisions was operating, the talking heads on a news channel soundlessly belittling the world's leaders. Bea ducked down and pulled out a pint of whiskey. Without asking, she poured two shots and thrust one across the bar.

"This'll warm your teeth from the inside out. Bottoms up and welcome home." Bea threw her own glass back like she meant it, the spirits gone before Charlotte decided if she could even stomach the stuff.

"Go on," Bea said. "For courage."

Charlotte raised the shot glass and sniffed. The smell slightly turned her stomach. She preferred craft beer and hadn't had whiskey since Sammy, her senior prom date, snuck a bottle into the gym. She took a meager sip, closed her eyes, and tipped her head. The spirit burned all the way down but had a redeeming cinnamon sweetness to it. A warmth crept up Charlotte's spine.

For courage.

"You're here about Chuck, huh? About damned time."

Charlotte bristled. She frowned at Bea and set the glass on the bar. Time was irrelevant; she'd had reasons for leaving, and she'd sure as hell had reasons for staying away.

"Your dad could have used your help months ago," Bea said.

14

Dropping from the barstool, Charlotte fished some bills from her purse and plunked a crumpled pile of ones next to her empty glass.

"Thank you, *Ms. Douglas.*" Charlotte turned toward the door. "I've got to go. I have a lot to deal with before I leave on Monday."

"Ah, now, honey, I told ya' to call me Bea. For eff's sake, I didn't mean nothin' by it." Bea's voice rose. "We're just worried about your daddy, is all. He's a good man. You're leavin'? On Monday? But today's Saturday. What you want to go and do that for, girl? Ya' just got here."

Charlotte paused, her hand gripping the doorframe. She was there to check the boxes and do her duty. That someone who watched her grow up and witnessed all the crap it entailed would judge *her*, instead of her father, was beyond comprehension.

"I knew I shouldn't have come."

"Charlie, I—"

"Stupid of me to do it anyway. And my name is *Charlotte*, Ms. Douglas. Thanks for the drink." Feeling the heat of Bea's stare between her shoulder blades, Charlotte quickly let herself out.

Everyone had always taken Chuck's side. Clearly, nothing had changed. Why would she ever think it could?

She turned and caught a glimpse of movement at the north end of the marina. A charter boat named the *Erie Mermaid* pulled into one of the farthest dock slips. Fishing poles stood guard off the stern, and contact information decorated the side. The man at the helm looked to be in his early thirties with a rusty beard and unruly blond hair, bleached nearly white. He stood at the wheel petting a dog in the captain's chair.

Charlotte grimaced. She missed Alfredo; he'd give her far more courage than whiskey.

The fisherman maneuvered next to the dock, and a teenager in a baseball cap scrambled from the cabin to the back of the boat and threw a line over the nearest pylon. The engine cut out, and the man leapt over the side and onto the dock with the dog at his heels. His efficiency of movement Charlotte had never mastered herself, after years of trying.

Nor would she *ever* master it. Nor did she care.

Not anymore.

She'd wasted enough time. The whiskey burning a hole in her gut, she glanced up at a small sign above the only remaining entrance—*The Lakeside Line.*

Straightening her shoulders, she grasped the handle and pushed with more force than necessary. The move proved anticlimactic and led to an empty hallway connecting the rear of The Surly Sturgeon to another door. It stood slightly ajar, and she could hear voices—her father's, for sure, and another man's.

Charlotte hurried forward, but her pace sputtered and stalled. At the entrance to the office, a vacant reception desk greeted her, its only ornamentation a thin film of dust and a dying, potted philodendron. Sunlight pierced through a glass-block window of a vacant adjoining office to the left. She shielded the glare with her hand and turned to her right.

Oh.

Chuck Sutton sat in an office chair at an ornate, mahogany table, likely a kitchen dining table in its previous life. Stacks of print issues spanned a third of the surface, and neat rows of sticky notes blanketed the remainder. Charlotte's father peered down at them as he listened to his cell phone on speaker.

"Chuck, I need some assurances my ad for the Pilgrims & Pastries event will make it into the next issue. I can't afford to have another slip-up with dates," a voice said. "Last time, we had people knocking on our door at all hours on a Sunday."

Chuck glanced at Charlotte. "Truly sorry about that, Michael. Entirely my fault." The note of confidence in his voice faded on the final word, leaving it more of a question than a statement. "I'll hit it out of the park for you, I promise. It won't happen again."

"Yeah, no problem. You're doing your best. Good thing October's Scares & Scones was a two-day affair, or we'd barely have made enough to pay for our advertising."

Silent, Chuck stared at his daughter, a look of confusion in his dark eyes so very like Charlotte's own.

Charlotte stared back.

Faint crow's feet highlighted Chuck's gaze, and his stomach had thickened a bit, but his shoulders were broad, and his muscular forearms could still power through a base hit. Most of his hair was as dark and wavy as hers, but there were flecks of silver and white now peppering his temples. Distinguished. He had aged, yes, but definitely not in a bad way. The past decade had been annoyingly kind.

Figures.

"You with me, Chuck?" The man on the line said.

Chuck's attention skittered away from Charlotte, and he turned back to his notes. "I'm sorry. What did you say? You're breaking up."

The customer repeated himself.

"Right." Chuck scanned a colorful square. He looked at Charlotte and down at the paper. "Truly sorry about that... Michael. Entirely my fault. It won't happen again."

"No problem. I'll hit you up in a couple of weeks about the December Jingles & Gingerbread thing." The caller hung up.

Chuck wrote a new note and crumpled the old one into a ball. With a practiced flick, he shot the wad overhand into a small basketball hoop hanging on the far wall. It ricocheted against the rim and dropped into the trash can beneath.

"Two points," Chuck said, as he always did. He turned toward his daughter. The look of confusion returned, and he thrust his hand across the table. "Chuck Sutton."

Charlotte sucked in a breath. Blinking, she allowed him to fold her sweaty palm into his dry, leathery one. Tears burned behind her closed eyelids.

"Please, have a seat."

Charlotte slumped into a chair.

"Can I help you with something?"

She hadn't known what to expect—coming home—but this was definitely not it. With a swipe of her cheek, she pointed to the high school graduation picture on the bookshelf above Chuck's head.

"It's me. Charlotte."

"Charlotte?" Chuck looked at the picture and back at his daughter. Comprehension flitted across his face. "Well, of course. Charlie. I was just..."

Chuck didn't finish his sentence.

My god. He didn't know who I was.

He didn't know.

3

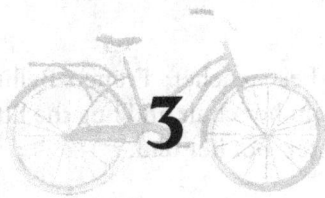

The sudden clatter of the door interrupted Charlotte's thoughts.

"I gave that bat-shit-crazy, beautiful old woman the rent check, Chuck. We're paid up for another month. Brews on the house."

"Oh, my gosh." Charlotte spun around. "Mr. B?"

Franco Bellimer, Charlotte's high school English and journalism teacher, stood in the doorway. The beer-keg-of-a-man, with thin arms and legs, could have passed for Bea's slightly younger brother. In his hands, he held two longnecks.

"Charlotte?" Bellimer's voice hushed, and he pushed the door closed with his shoulder. "Bea said you were home, but, well, my goodness. It's really you."

Favorite student and favorite teacher faced each other. Charlotte's heart raced, then slowed. It would be all right. Mr. B had always made *everything* right.

"All grown up and a lovelier sight I've never seen." Bellimer smiled. "And a published writer, to boot. I'm so proud of you."

Chuck remained silent.

"It's great to see you, Mr. B. Doesn't look like you've changed a bit." His reading glasses still defied gravity at the very tip of his nose, and he wore an obligatory tweed sport coat with elbow patches—one Charlotte was almost certain she'd seen before.

Franco Bellimer rubbed his head, then patted his stomach. "A lot balder. A little fatter." He chuckled and tapped his temple. "Ah, but also a little wiser, Miss Sutton. So, there's that. Time is the best teacher, I always say."

"Deep, Mr. B."

Time wasn't the best teacher; Franco Bellimer was. Charlotte wanted to leap up from her chair and hug the little man. He was the reason she was a writer, not her dad.

Never her dad.

She hadn't thought she'd ever be as good of a writer as Chuck, but Mr. B had taught her to trust her instincts—to believe in herself.

Bellimer dangled one of the beers in Chuck's direction. "Brew?"

"You go ahead," Chuck mumbled.

"Charlotte?" Bellimer said. "Seems to me you're well past drinking age."

"Thanks. I'd love one." Charlotte grabbed the offering and guzzled about half the contents. She was grateful for something to do with her hands and equally grateful for something to do with her mouth. Anything had to be better than talking about fathers who no longer recognized their daughters.

"So, this is typical?" Charlotte lifted the bottle she clung to like a life preserver. Her fingernail tapped the glass, seeking the corner of the label to peel. "Free brew from The Surly Sturgeon?"

Bellimer nodded. "Honestly, it's no wonder the marina is hanging on by a fishhook. Bea gives away far more drink than she sells."

Charlotte motioned to the office. "Are you part of all this, then?"

"I started working for your dad about three years ago, just after I retired from teaching."

"Most days, I couldn't put the paper together without Franco."

Chuck picked up one of his notes—his finger saving its place. He read it. Tacked it down again. Picked up another. Read it. Put it down.

Charlotte shrugged. "I, um—"

"It's great to see your daughter, Chuck," Bellimer said, tipping his beer in Charlotte's direction. "She's sure grown up, hasn't she?"

"Yes, of course." Chuck fidgeted with a note and faced Charlotte, fully, for the first time. "But why did you come?"

Why, indeed?

"Somebody named Jake called." Charlotte swallowed, only able to muster a whisper. "He said you might be having some health issues."

Chuck smiled. "Jake's a good boy—a friend who always steps up to the plate when I need him."

A team player. Spectacular.

"How *is* your health?"

"Not as good as yours, I'm sure, but no need to bother with that right now." Chuck laughed it off, his confusion replaced by a familiar confidence. Charlotte wasn't 100% convinced.

"Stand up, kid, so I can really see what you're all about." Her father grabbed her hand and rose, pulling her up with him.

Straight and tall, Chuck capped out only a few inches above her. Charlotte tried not to slouch, feeling like a giraffe in a cage viewed with judgement by the zookeeper. Old habits were hard to break. Growing up, she'd hated her height, her hair, her flat-as-Stanley chest. She'd been insecure about how her father, and everyone, perceived her. She could not help it.

"She's the mirror of you, Chuck." Bellimer took a sip from his beer.

"She certainly is." Chuck grinned. "A might prettier, though, I'd say. A beauty."

"Sure is." Bellimer raised his bottle and saluted his former student.

Charlotte considered bolting for the door.

"Welcome home, Charlie," Chuck said, "even if it took your old man being down to his last out to get you here. Sure glad Jake put through that call. Meant to do it myself, of course, but I've been busy. I never quite found the time."

Bullshit.

Chuck beamed, motioning for his daughter to take her seat. "We've got a lot to talk about."

"That's my cue to head home." Bellimer stood. "You need anything before I go?"

"Nope. Got my Charlie here. Teamwork makes the dream work, I always say."

Charlotte rolled her eyes at Bellimer. Her father obviously still loved his sports clichés.

"We'll catch up later, Charlotte," Bellimer said. "I'd love to treat you to dinner."

Charlotte shook her head. "I'm only here for a couple of days, Mr. B. I have to get back to Pittsburgh."

"I'm sorry to hear that." He sandwiched Charlotte's hands between his own. "For so many reasons. I wish you could stick around for a bit."

"Thanks, but I... I can't."

Bellimer nodded. "If not dinner, could I at least steal you for another beer at the bar? We've got a lot to talk about, too. Quite a lot." He threw a pointed look at her father. "But I'll try to keep it short. Promise. Just a drink is all I'm asking."

"Um, sure. Tomorrow night?"

"Perfect. Stop by the Sturgeon around game time. I'll plan on it."

Franco Bellimer patted her on the shoulder and was out the door in a lick.

Deserter.

Charlotte's unease returned with the silence left in his wake. She slowly faced Chuck.

"Yeah. So, Mr. B is awesome," she said, at a loss for anything else.

"Yes. Yes, he is." Chuck slumped in his chair and rubbed his temples. "He's been a great deal of help to me. I couldn't keep this paper alive without him, especially now."

"Oh."

Chuck tipped back, his attention now fully on his daughter. "So, how long has it been since you visited Lakeside? Five years? Six? I can't remember the last—"

"I haven't been back since high school graduation," Charlotte said. "Why would you even think I had?"

Chuck cocked his head. "Fair point. I just assumed you might have been up to see your high school buddies and didn't tell me."

Charlotte shook her head. "I didn't have high school buddies—just Sammy, and we kind of lost touch after graduation."

"Sammy bought the House of Beauty a few years back. He calls it Clippers now, I think."

"The hair salon? That's fantastic."

"You should stop in and see him," Chuck said. "If you have the time."

"I should try."

But she probably wouldn't.

"I'd love to see Sammy. It's been so long."

"A little warning, though," Chuck said. "You might get a bit of a chilly reception."

"What do you mean?"

Chuck shrugged. "You were best friends, weren't you, kid? For the longest time, your mom and I thought you might end up marrying that boy. When you left, he didn't take it very well. I bump into him every now and then. He always used to ask about you. Over the years, he's stopped asking. I think he was angry you didn't stay in contact."

23

"Angry at me?" Charlotte shook her head. "Nah. It's Sammy from Miami. Mr. Chill. Sammy never gets angry at anyone."

"As you say."

Charlotte shrugged. "It *would* be nice to see him again. I miss Sammy. But I really won't have time. I have to get back to—"

"Pittsburgh... you said." Chuck shifted. He looked at the notes lining his table. "Seems like a waste to drive all the way up here and leave so soon."

"I've got a job at an ad agency downtown," Charlotte said. "It's part-time, but I don't want to screw it up. I'm hoping to go full-time soon."

"Right." Chuck nodded. "Congratulations."

"Thanks."

Seconds passed. The silence left Charlotte parched and on the verge of tears. Chuck tapped one of his many notes, plucked it up, read it, and placed it meticulously back in its spot.

"There *is* another option," he said, finally. "You could work here at the newspaper."

"What?"

"I could use another writer."

"You can't be serious. What purpose would that serve?" Charlotte squinted at her father. What was his goal? How would it benefit him, exactly?

Chuck glanced down at the table and out the window again. In profile, he looked older—drawn—as if he'd aged just since she'd walked through the door. Charlotte allowed the silence to grow, unwilling to be the one to break it.

Chuck turned back to Charlotte. "Look, kid, we both know I wasn't around much when you were growing up, and I'd like to spend some time with you. Get to know you better, if you'll let me."

Right.

"What would be the point, Chuck? I'm not going to be here long enough for either of us to bother trying."

Chuck's lips clenched to a rigid line.

Had she gone too far?

He rolled his chair back a few feet from the table and propped an ankle on the opposite knee. "Get straight to the point, don't you, kid? Line drive right down the middle. Good to hear you speak your piece, I guess."

Charlotte shrugged. "I'm serious. Why would you want me to stay? You didn't even call me to come. Jake did."

"You're right." Chuck nodded. "I should have called. You're here now, though. The way I see it, you came home when you weren't expected to. That's a start."

"What's the punchline?"

"No punchline." Chuck shrugged. "Jake was right, though. My health is... a bit off, right now, is all. You'd be helping me out while the doctor gets my issues figured out. Why not stay for a couple of weeks? What's the harm? It would give us a chance to spend some time together, and you could visit with Franco and Sammy and anyone else you'd like to look up from back in the day. Stay, why don't you?"

Why don't I?

The question confused her. Turning away, Charlotte roamed the room, seeking answers and, instead, finding a shelf full of classics. Chuck had collected beautifully bound titles from Shakespeare, Twain, Orwell, Hemingway, and the like, for as long as she could remember. She scanned the well-worn spines, barely seeing through a film of tears fighting to break free. She'd given some of the books to him as birthday or Father's Day or Christmas gifts. He loved his old books.

Charlotte shook her head. What possible good could come of staying? They'd never be close. Not like a father and daughter should be. Too much time had passed. She wasn't sure what she could have done differently to have a real father-daughter relationship.

Or that she still even *wanted* one.

"What do you say, kid?"

She tipped back the bitter dregs of lukewarm beer, wishing she could bolt to The Surly Sturgeon and get another. With a sigh, she met her father's steady gaze.

"I'm 28 years old, and you barely know me." Charlotte's voice came out a croak. "That's what I say."

Chuck blinked. "True. And you barely know me, but every game is game seven."

"Not for me, remember? I sucked at sports. And you hardly ever came to my games, anyway." Charlotte's voice rose, sounding loud in her own ears. Whiny. Mean.

She didn't care.

Charlotte allowed the tension, building to a fever pitch over the course of nearly twelve hours, to flood her brain and come out her mouth.

"I always felt like you were punishing me for something I did wrong. Or was it because I *couldn't* do something? Because I wasn't good enough at sports?"

"What? Of course, not." Chuck leaned forward and gripped the table. His knuckles bled white. "Dear, God, Charlie, how could you even think that?"

"What else should I think?" Charlotte shrugged.

"If that's truly what you believe, it's my biggest regret."

"There was a lot to regret. Take your pick."

Chuck frowned. "I didn't care if you were any good at sports or if you even played. I just wanted something we could have in common... something we could enjoy together."

"Then why didn't you come to my games?"

Chuck sighed. "I was trying to keep the peace. That was a whole lot easier when I wasn't around. I can't explain it any better. When you were little, I'd roll a ball to you in the grass for hours, and you'd laugh and laugh and roll it back. When you got older, your mom played dress-up and bought you dolls and braided your hair. I just wanted to teach you how to throw a slider. Sports was all I knew.

It was all I could bring to the table. Girls were a complete mystery to me." Chuck's voice lowered. "Heck, if I'd understood the female mind a bit better, Elise and I might never have gotten married in the first place."

"How could you say that?" The heat of anger built again, threatening to overwhelm Charlotte. "It wasn't just the sports. You missed my high school *and* college graduations. Dads don't do that. Not if they give a shit."

"You don't think I didn't feel bad about that?" Chuck shook his head. "I was on tour. My writing paid for us to live. It paid for you to *go* to college. Come on, kid, I'm not saying that's a reason to miss the big things in your life, but it does explain it a little."

Charlotte frowned. "Sounds to me like you are trying to justify it to yourself."

Chuck's guttural laugh was hollow, devoid of humor. "Maybe I am. Look, I'm running out of time, and you're my daughter. I wish you'd stay a while. That's all there is to it. There are a lot of things you don't know about me, and your mother, and what led to our divorce. Truly, Charlie, for the sake of the legacy I leave my family... the newspaper, cottage, everything—"

The outer door banged, and footsteps echoed in the hall. A fleeting panic stole across Chuck's face.

"Charlie, there's so much I've needed to tell you."

The dog from the fishing charter boat, a shepherd of some kind, bounded into the room. Its nails skittered *click, click, click* across the cement floor. It skidded to a stop at the sight of Charlotte, and backed up a couple of feet.

"Well, hello, beautiful," Charlotte said.

The dog, a welcome distraction, had no tail to wag. Its nubbed behind wiggled at a furious pace, and the pup curled around and returned to the doorway.

Charlotte wanted to wrap her arms around it. Its coat of mottled rust and white, with splashes of gold and a solid white ruff around its neck, reminded her of a Jackson Pollock painting. She reached out her hand, palm up.

"Where're you going, floof? Who's a good dog? Are you a good boy or a good girl? Can't tell under all that hair. Do you like scritches?"

The dog lay down on its stomach, creeping a foot closer. One brown eye and one blue eye focused on Charlotte.

Chuck's voice rose. "There's so much you don't know. I need to explain some things. You don't—"

Charlotte registered more movement at the door.

"Hey, Dad, Jake and I caught the biggest walleye yet." The teenager from the boat burst through the doorway and came to an abrupt halt, shepherd-like, when he saw Charlotte, his face looking as startled as hers must. He was tall. The Cleveland baseball hat did nothing to hide the dark, wavy hair a bit longer than Charlotte's own pixie cut, and a smattering of Charlotte's freckles crossed the bridge of his nose. Unlike Charlotte, he held himself with a natural grace, and his skin was as brown as Charlotte's was pale. Behind him stood the fisherman from the *Erie Mermaid*.

Charlotte whirled to face her father. "Seriously?"

"Charlie, I—"

Charlotte threw her hand up and hurried toward the door. The dog barked, and the man and the boy parted to let her pass. Gasping, she barreled into the outer hallway.

"Dad, was that Charlotte?"

The young voice sounded just like her father's.

A knife twisted in Charlotte's chest again and again and again.

28

4

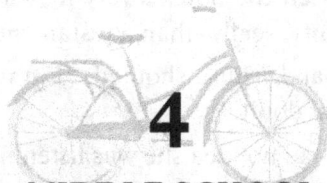

MIDDLE SCHOOL

Twelve-year-old Charlotte pulled the hoodie up over her ears, to no avail. She could still hear the shouting coming from the kitchen below.

"Would it kill you?" Elise Sutton said. "There are only so many games in the season, and I told you I couldn't make it. You signed her up for the damned team in the first place. Why don't you go to her games? She's your daughter. I mean, really, would it kill you?"

"Easy, El." Chuck's mellow voice, the opposite of Mom's, was almost too low to hear. "They threw me a signing party, and then my flight was delayed. I got here as fast as I could. Charlie will understand."

Her father's murmurings, and the use of his boyish nickname for her, hung around Charlotte's neck like a participation medal. Her stomach clenched. She was why her parents fought so much, and she hated being in the middle of it. It was hard not to take sides when Chuck never made it to her games. Or anything else. He had stuff to do for his book.

Big, important stuff.

He was a big, important author, according to her mother. Thinks he's all that, according to her mother. Not to mention the damned chippy assistant with a tight ass and perky boobs, according to her mother.

TMI, Mom.

Since Charlotte could remember, her parents had slept in separate bedrooms, and they never held hands. Chuck kissed Elise on the cheek before he left the house every morning, but it served as more of a ritual—a duty, really—than a testament to their love.

"Be a shitty husband," Elise shouted. "I'm used to it. Just don't be a shitty father. Just don't."

Thank God they had no idea she was listening, or it would make things worse. Charlotte had feigned a migraine three-quarters of the way through her personal hell—sitting the bench at the seventh-grade Bay Area Biting Walleyes girls' basketball game. Neither parent had attended and witnessed the embarrassment; she'd beaten them home. They thought she'd gone to a team pizza party with her friends after the win—about as likely as Charlotte needing a B-cup-size bra anytime soon.

Slim. Flat-as-Stanley slim.

Charlotte didn't actually have friends. Or boobs.

What sport would Chuck have her bomb next? He'd started her on little league softball, of course. Charlotte had ended up in tears, afraid to leave the dugout. Then volleyball, which hadn't gone well either. The coach, *obviously* holding a grudge against humanity and pre-teenage girls, had told Charlotte she was incapable of walking and chewing gum at the same time. The coach had demanded she stand beside the net until a more athletic teammate set the ball right to her. Stand there and wait, he'd said, until it comes to you. Then tap the ball over.

Wait and tap.

The instructions had sounded simple—easy, even—but Charlotte's eye-hand coordination had been as much of a bust as the walking-and-chewing-gum thing. She wished she'd gotten points for trying.

Chuck's unfailing optimism that some sport—any sport—would eventually stick just made it worse. It was never going to happen, no matter how much her father wanted it to. Maybe it was *best* he missed her games. Enduring the humiliation was bad enough. Far worse when her father witnessed it.

"Why the hell didn't you call her? Wish her luck?" Elise rattled around in the cupboards, finding the noisiest pans to bang. "Seriously, Chuck, what's so hard? She just needs to know you care. Do you? Do you care about either of us?"

Charlotte winced.

"Of course, I care. Look, I'm not exactly batting a thousand here. I don't know what to talk about with a 12-year-old girl, is all," Chuck said. "I don't understand her. It would have been easier if we'd had a son. Maybe when she's older, we'll have more in common."

Not your son, Chuck. And there's nothing I can do about it.

"She's not a boy! She's never going to *be* a boy. She's not some kid you can build a team around!"

Mom was just getting started. Charlotte considered climbing down the tree outside her window and walking through the front door to put an end to the brawl, but her presence had never stopped her parents in the past. She could write the script on how the fight would progress. Chuck would remain calm like he always did—listen but not engage during Elise's expletive-peppered bitch out. His silence would only make her mother angrier. She'd say the same thing again and again in a slightly different way, as if she could wear down Chuck with repetition alone. At some point, Chuck would completely tune her out. Or tease her.

Or both.

"She's not a boy." Elise's voice rose to a screech. "Dammit, Chuck. You listening to me? You aren't even listening to me, are you?"

Chuck snorted. "Come on, hon. Relax."

Please. You'll only make it worse. Please don't.

"You're cute when you're mad, Elise, but there's no reason to get so fired up." Chuck's snort turned to laughter.

"You sonofabitch." Elise gasped, a wounded howl of a sound. "Cute? Don't you call me cute. Don't you dare call me cute. Stop laughing at me! You bet I'm fired up. I'm totally fired up!"

Her mother's thick mascara would be running down her cheeks in inky streams by now. Her face red. Her chest heaving. Her bleached hair whipping around her cheeks, sticking to the tears.

The argument was no longer about Charlotte.

"Fired up? Lord, woman, that's an understatement." Chuck laughed harder. "My Barbie with attitude."

Charlotte threw on a coat and gloves. She yanked her journal from between her mattress and box springs and grabbed a pencil from her desk.

"Get the hell out." Elise's high voice ricocheted off the thin, cottage walls. "Get out!"

"Come on, hon, seriously—"

"I mean it, you bastard. Don't you ever call me that! You want attitude? I'll give you attitude. Get out and don't come back!"

Classic. Sutton. Shitstorm.

Hurrying out onto her second-story porch, Charlotte was just in time to feel and hear the slamming of the front door below her. Her father didn't look up as he took off down the path, his shoulders slumped and his gait slow and steady.

He'd go to the bar and come back after dinner. And her mother would let him. Her crazy-assed mother would let him, even if he was drunk.

Shaking, she turned her attention to the expanse of Lake Erie. It had been an unseasonably warm winter, the temperatures only falling below freezing a couple of times since December. The water looked deceptively calm with no sign of ice. With a deep breath, she sought peace in the blue-black surface and let her heart begin to return to a normal rhythm.

She pulled the strings of her hoodie, tucking a long chunk of hair under the fabric and allowing her mouth and nose to feel the crisp air. Hunching down on a wooden rocker her mother had rocked her to sleep in when she was a baby, Charlotte took a swipe at her moist cheek, opened her journal, and flipped to a blank page.

5

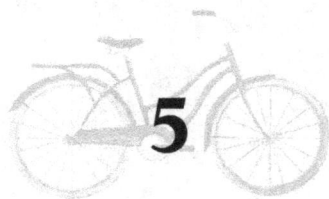

Great hacking sobs poured from Charlotte as she ran from the newspaper office. Chuck could as easily have raised a baseball bat, slicing it through the air again and again to shatter her heart into pieces she'd never be able to glue back together.

She paused on the waterfront path. There'd be no time to walk on the dock. She'd go back to Pittsburgh. Even if she left immediately, she'd have to get a hotel room somewhere. She was too upset to drive the nearly three and a half hours, and there was the matter of eating, something she hadn't done since the drive-thru on her way north—the breakfast sandwich sitting like a worried lump in her stomach for hours.

As she approached Sutton's Choice, Charlotte couldn't quite grasp what had just happened. How could her father have not told her he had a son? How old was her brother? What was his name?

Charlie?

No. Damn. Way. It had better not be Charlie.

I bet it's Charlie.

Who was his mother? Did Elise know? Had Chuck re-married? So many questions.

Charlotte hurried onto the front porch. She looked to the lake, pleading with her watery friend to cough up some answers and heal her, as it had done so many times before. Nothing but hurt rose to the surface. She'd learned to swim in Lake Erie. To fish. To sail. Since birth, her soul had been tied to the water, at peace with the water.

Until now.

Peace eluded her. Answers eluded her.

"Never, ever again," she muttered.

No longer giving a damn if she should or should not let herself in, Charlotte opened the front door of Sutton's Choice. The cottage was small and drafty, and the floors weren't exactly plumb, but she found strength in its dusty corners. It had sturdily withstood more than one hundred years of Northeasters and more than 14 years of her parents' constant bickering.

Her father, with his baseball pension and endorsements and book deals, could have bought a cottage three times the size, but had chosen to remain in the family home, humble as it was. The furniture, shabby-chic from the days of her mother collecting hand-me-downs at yard sales, looked exactly as it had when Charlotte was young. The small living room featured the only hint of modern upgrades—a big-screen TV and leather recliner for watching sports.

She crept up the stairs, avoiding the squeaky treads that could have alerted Chuck and Elise dozens of times that she was coming home late from Sammy's.

To the left. Step. Step. Right. Step. Left. Left. Left.

A literal step back in time.

Natural as breathing, Charlotte skipped the second stair from the top. It should have been ripped out and replaced by now, it was so noisy. She stopped on the landing. The first door led to the largest room where she assumed her father still slept. She didn't bother to confirm it. A spare bedroom and bath beckoned at the end of the hall. On the left, she opened the door to her old bedroom and came up short. The walls of the small space had been painted a deep navy blue, a drastic change from her favorite pale violet. Cleveland baseball memorabilia plastered every surface.

Shit.

The boy had replaced her.

For a teenager's room, it was surprisingly neat. A framed picture of a young Chuck dressed in his baseball uniform graced a nearby dresser. Next to it sat a picture of Chuck's son, also in a uniform.

The room served as the boy's shrine to baseball.

Damned baseball.

Or the boy's shrine to his father.

Feeling the blue walls folding in on her, Charlotte stepped past the twin bed with a baseball-shaped throw pillow at its foot and opened the door to the upstairs porch. It was bare of furniture but for her mother's old rocker, in which Charlotte had sat and written in her journal almost every day as a child. Though unprotected from the elements, its arms were oiled to a sheen. Charlotte dropped down into it. The weathered wood engulfed her, cradled her. In that moment, she allowed everything to fully sink in.

She had a brother.

Chuck hadn't told her.

Charlotte stared out at the waterfront dock. The cement slab, nearly the length of a football field, shot out into the blackness of Lake Erie. Two smaller docks branched to the left of the main dock. Water sprayed up and over the furthest, its liquid tentacles creeping across the L-shaped arm and seeping back into the depths.

It was Lake Erie she would miss. Nothing more.

She'd never be back, and there was no reason to stick around another minute longer. Charlotte grabbed the rocker, light but unwieldy, and wrestled it through the door into the boy's room. She set it down long enough to adjust the baseball pillow, just so, against the headboard. Smoothing the wrinkles from the bedspread, she hefted the rocker and turned toward the door.

Good luck, kid. You'll need it.

Dampening the ungracious thought, she hurried toward the stairs. There was no reason to visit the other second-floor rooms. She no longer cared. Sutton's Choice had been her childhood home and her prison—a prison she was again breaking out of once and for all. She took the rocker downstairs and out the back. With a flick of her keychain, she unlocked the hatch of her car and wrangled the seats into a flat position. Just as she was struggling to maneuver the pilfered memento into the back, tanned hands reached beyond hers and grasped the wood.

"Can I help you with that?"

The fisherman from the charter boat took the rocker from Charlotte's limp fingers. He lowered it to the gravel. A blur of red and white and gold flew past, leapt into the back of the car, and jumped into the front seat.

"Ah, hell. Come, Sydney."

Her new co-pilot was the dog from the office. They appeared to share a common goal—escaping Lakeside.

"Sydney, here." The voice was firm, not angry.

The dog jumped out of the car, keeping its intent gaze trained on its master. The man pulled a treat from his pocket and gave a simple hand motion. The dog sat.

"Good girl." The man turned toward Charlotte. "Sorry about that. She loves a car ride."

Charlotte shrugged.

Frowning, he dipped his chin. "You're leaving, then."

It was not a question; Charlotte nodded anyway.

"I'm Jake Forrester. I left you the message about Chuck's health."

Charlotte sucked in a breath. "Yeah? Thanks. Reeeeealllly appreciate that."

"I'm sorry," Jake said. "I didn't realize your dad never told you about your brother. Can you please—"

"No. No, I cannot."

Charlotte yanked the rocker from the ground and heaved it into her car, nearly taking out a window. Jake sighed as she shut the hatch. She paid him no mind, though it was difficult. After years of looking down at men, she felt somewhat dwarfed by this one. She opened the driver's side door and collapsed onto the seat. As she began to pull the door shut, Jake blocked it with his forearm, the strength obvious through the long-sleeved shirt he wore beneath his fishing vest.

"I totally get why you are upset, but you can't leave," Jake said.

Charlotte looked him full in the face. "Not to be rude, but watch me."

"Your dad isn't well. Please, can we talk about this?"

Charlotte's hands gripped the wheel at 10 and two. She faced forward, staring at the back of her family home. The flowerbeds near the steps needed weeding, something her mother had always enjoyed. Chuck didn't appear to have a green thumb.

Nor, apparently, did his son.

"Why didn't he tell me?"

"Honestly? I don't know." Jake paused. "It's a question I don't have a full answer to. I'm willing to tell you what I do know, though, if you're willing to listen." He offered his hand, palm up. "How about a walk on the dock to cool down, and then we can talk about it? Have you eaten today? Bea does a great lobster bisque."

The guy sounded like a crisis counselor—defuse and compromise. Charlotte glanced at his hand. Strong and tanned, it was the hand of a worker. His blue eyes hosted pale eyelashes and a hint of laugh lines. His neatly trimmed beard framed a hesitant smile.

He looked honest enough, well-meaning.

Charlotte's gut rolled with acid, wanting answers and food and maybe another shot of whiskey, all at the same time. She glanced down. Sydney stared up at her. The dog's tongue lolled to the side, as she waited as patiently as her owner for Charlotte's decision.

"Fine." Grumbling, Charlotte ignored Jake's hand and stepped from the car. "Fine."

It wasn't.

She shut the door and leaned against it. No doubt, she'd regret caving to his offer.

Scratch that.

She already did.

* * * * *

Charlotte dragged her jacket closed, tying her belt and pulling the hood up. From the look of the waves still cresting on the dock, it would be windier out near the flagpole standing guard at the very end. She and Sammy had spent many nights there, counting boat lights on the water and dodging walls of midges, so as not to get any of the flying insects stuck in their ice cream cones.

Sydney, off leash, never strayed more than a couple of yards away. Jake walked stride-for-stride beside Charlotte. Now that he had gotten her out of the car, he seemed in no hurry to engage. They were just out for a companionable stroll about Lakeside, much like any of the thousands of vacationers who swarmed the community in the warmest of months.

Charlotte had grown up watching the leaves turn color in October, the fall of snow on barren branches in January, the emerging buds of the cottonwoods in May—the Lakeside miracles of nature most summer vacationers never experienced. They were only around for the mid-summer heat, burgeoning gardens, shuffleboard tournaments, and sailing regattas—the grounds neat and orderly, the special events planned down to the minutest of detail.

June, July, and early August saw the largest percentage of visitors. In the off-season, after the gates went up and the party ended, Lakeside took off her perfectly ruffled skirts, removed her makeup, and let her hair down. It was as if the little town and its waterfront had two faces—the genteel, perfectly made-up summer lady of bygone days and a raw, unkempt woman the other nine months of the year.

To Charlotte, the latter was more interesting. More real.

She pulled a step ahead of Jake and stopped near the empty boat racks. The waterfront was stripped of its nautical adornments except for a couple of kayaks lying on the pebbled shore. She glanced at Jake. His hands were thrust into his pockets, his chin tilted into the wind.

Perhaps, the fisherman had the gift of patience.

Charlotte, on the other hand, had none.

"Look, I'm sorry," she said, breaking the silence. "It's not your fault Chuck makes me lose my shit. I don't like surprises, and I shouldn't have taken it out on you."

"Apology unnecessary but accepted." Jake nodded. "I can see why you'd be upset. Finding out you have a brother is a heck of a surprise."

"Half-brother. How long have you known my esteemed father, anyway?"

Jake picked up an abandoned plastic bottle and placed it in a nearby recycling bin. He motioned her toward the pavilion. "About seven years. I met him after I graduated from college and moved up here to work on the algae bloom issue."

"I see."

They passed the stairs to the upper deck of the pavilion and stepped beneath the arched entrance leading onto the cement dock. The Lake Erie water level was higher than average. Rope swayed across the cement from pylon to pylon, bearing a sign reading "Dock Closed"—an illusion of prevention in case an off-season walker fell into the drink.

The pavilion businesses, closed after the season, presented dark storefronts. The sight of a stray "I Love Lakeside" t-shirt, hanging lopsided on a hanger in a window, saddened Charlotte for no apparent reason. During the summer, she might have seen toddlers splashing in the kiddie pool to the right of the dock or a family creating a sand sculpture on the beach at the base of the sailing club.

But no one was here in the fall. No one would know or care that she'd returned to Lakeside and gone again.

As if I never existed.

"I'm a marine biologist," Jake added. "After I got my master's and the grant for my project ran out, I decided to stick around. Bea lets me use the apartment above the restaurant, as long as I help her with things at the marina. It's a pretty good gig."

"You're in the apartment Chuck rented after my parents' divorce?"

"Oh, yeah," Jake said. "Yeah, that's the one, all right. Sorry to bring it up."

"Apology unnecessary but accepted."

"Thanks." Jake offered a low chuckle. "I stayed because I really love being on the water. The fishing is fantastic here."

"I know. I grew up here."

"Of course. I love Lakeside, and the people too. Your dad helped me get to know everyone. He's been a great friend."

"Mom called him Good-time Charlie. Chuck has always had plenty of friends." The envy Charlotte recognized in her voice angered her, made her feel weak. "I didn't. I never really fit in."

The previous spring, she'd received a Bay Area High School class reunion invitation. She'd thrown it in the trash. Unlike her father, she'd been the local outcast—a nobody—and couldn't possibly have gained any ground in the ten years since her departure.

With the exception of Sammy, her peers hadn't made her feel welcome. Her social standing had suffered further after she tripped a teammate during a basketball game and her nearly six-foot frame landed in a tangled pile of arms and legs to the chorus of "Timmmberrrr." Charlotte grimaced. Her classmates had dubbed her "The Tree," a far worse nickname than "Charlie," truth be told.

And here she was. The Tree had come home, would be leaving again for the last time, and no one was around to care.

"As a biologist, what's your expert opinion? If a tree falls in the woods and no one hears it, does it really make a sound?"

Jake slowed. "Um, I don't—"

"Forget it," Charlotte said. "Inside joke."

No one would be impacted by her Lakeside comings and goings. Her presence, or lack thereof, made no difference. Quite the opposite, if it were Chuck leaving, the town would throw a damned farewell parade.

"The cottonwoods are really beautiful in the spring," Jake said. "I hope they never get taken out in a storm. We had a lot of downed trees about a month ago. Serious Northeaster."

His awkward attempt to lead the conversation back toward neutral waters somewhat humored Charlotte, though for the wrong reasons. She was being handled like a fireworks display—with an overly gentle touch and a healthy fear of premature explosion. Perhaps his reaction was warranted.

"Sydney is beautiful," Charlotte said, cutting him a break. "May I pet... her, right?"

"Sure," Jake said.

Charlotte reached down, palm up. "Hi, pretty girl."

Sydney took her time about it, but eventually gave a sniff. Then a lick. Charlotte's hand brushed over the dog's head.

"Oh, you are beautiful, aren't you? And so soft." Charlotte's fingers sank into the fur at the animal's neck. The dog looked up and pulled back her lips, baring teeth.

Charlotte yanked her hand back. "Oh—"

Jake laughed. "It's okay. Really. She's smiling at you. Ferocious looking, huh? I taught her to do that when she was just a puppy, and she's been doing it ever since—usually when she's really glad to see me. I'm surprised she did it for you, though. She's not normally so comfortable with strangers. I think she likes you."

"Huh, well as long as she won't take off a finger."

Jake shrugged. "Not unless I tell her to."

"Comforting." Charlotte hesitated and, again, reached down to the dog. Sydney immediately pressed her weight against Charlotte's legs. "I've never seen this kind of coat. What is she? A mix?"

"She's an Aussie. An Australian shepherd. They come in all

colors, but she's a red merle. My family always had Aussies when I was a kid. They herded the sheep on our farm. Smartest dogs ever."

"Interesting."

"She loves being on the boat, too."

"I bet." Sydney suddenly dodged off, her focus on chasing a squirrel up a nearby tree. "Too bad you can't get her to herd fish."

"That would be something." There was an odd edge to Jake's voice, as if he were biting back what he didn't want to let go. "So, um, why didn't you respond to my calls? We were afraid Chuck didn't have your correct number for emergencies. I found your info on one of the notes on his desk when he started having problems."

Now we're getting to it.

Charlotte stopped near the lip of the cement. She glared down at the murky water, thick with foam and seaweed. She didn't answer Jake's question, deciding to parlay with her own.

"Why didn't my father come to my games? My birthday parties? My college graduation? Pointless questions, obviously. Sorry, but seeing your 419 number on my screen just reminded me of my childhood. Chuck wasn't around much. Too busy being the big-time author and partying with his fans."

"I see."

"Do you? Honestly? I don't even know why I'm here. I'm not the person to call in an emergency. My father is barely an acquaintance. I lived under the same roof with him, but I never really knew him, and he never really knew me. I'm over it."

"It doesn't *sound* like you are."

"I *am*," Charlotte snapped. "I don't owe him a damn thing."

"Whoa." Jake stepped back. "I didn't say you did."

"There was a time when I would have begged for a call from a 419 area code. Not anymore. I didn't return your call because there's no reason for anyone from here to be contacting me. Chuck is not my problem."

The silence between them, deafening, draped around Charlotte's shoulders, chilling her like no wind off the water would ever do.

"Crap. I'm sorry," she muttered, pulling in air. "Again. That was over the line."

"It's okay."

"He just makes me so mad."

Jake nodded. "I can see that."

Taking another deep breath, Charlotte pulled gloves from her pocket. "Yeah. So, I need to go to the end of the dock and circle the flagpole. It's tradition."

Jake nodded. "I'm in."

"You don't have to. It'll be my last time, and I'd like to say goodbye to the lake." Heat rose to Charlotte's chilled face. "Alone. I know that sounds ridiculous."

"It doesn't." Jake swept a hand in the direction of the flagpole. "You do you."

"Thank you." Charlotte threw a leg over the "Dock Closed" sign and put distance between them. She was vaguely aware of Sydney trotting along beside her. Dozens of seagulls dotted the wet pavement, taking full advantage of the lack of summer sunbathers keeping them from their favorite perch. With a *keow keow keow*, they rose in droves and took to the air as the Aussie swept through them. Charlotte's steps and heartbeat slowed. She reached the halfway mark, then three-quarters. Breathing easier, she ran her gloved hand, a familiar caress, around the flagpole and paused beneath the Lakeside beacon. Stepping forward, she tapped the northernmost edge of the cement with the toe of her shoe, like she'd done for almost three decades. The end of the dock was her Camelot, her place of tranquility.

It was a gray day. Charlotte's gaze sought Kelleys Island to the north—mere bumps and lumps of darkness on the horizon. To the left, even further away, Put-in-Bay beckoned with its pillared Perry's Monument. In a motorboat, it would take only about 20 minutes to cross over to the island, with its mile-long bar and golf carts attracting bridal parties, divorcees, and retirees looking for their spent youth beneath a sandy tiki hut. Chuck had been a regular there. Charlotte could only imagine how many women he'd picked up on a Saturday night. She assumed he still had his motorboat, but maybe not.

We all make choices. He made his, and I'll make mine.

With a final glance north, Charlotte ducked her head and began walking back to where Jake waited. Sydney bounded ahead, sending another gaggle of squawking seagulls to the clouds, and ran two rotations around her master's legs before stopping in front of him. He gave her a pat, and she accepted a treat.

Charlotte had been pretty hard on Jake, but it appeared he could take it. She'd likely owe him another apology, at some point. No doubt. It was that kind of day.

But she wouldn't leave.

Not just yet.

Charlotte pressed her chin against her zipper and braced her shoulders.

She needed answers.

She *deserved* answers.

And if Jake couldn't provide them, Chuck would have to.

6

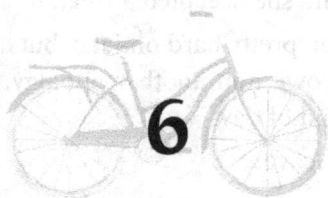

At The Surly Sturgeon, Jake gave a silent hand command to Sydney, who promptly lay down at Charlotte's feet.

"Good dog. Stay."

"Bea doesn't care if you've got her in here? Aren't there rules about that?"

"Nah. In a pinch, she makes one hell of a guard dog. We call her the surly bouncer."

"I see." Charlotte didn't.

It was the second time in just a few hours she found herself in The Surly Sturgeon. Yet, the dungeon-like space shone brighter than it had earlier in the day. Dozens of neon liquor signs blinked on every wall, and orange and white string lights—ode to the Cleveland Browns—framed every window facing the lake. Stained-glass pub shades hung above each table, throwing a shifting red, green, and amber glow onto white placemats printed with local business cards of funeral homes, bankers, and charter boats. With a fingertip, Charlotte traced the lettering of a card advertising "Buy Brew, Get 2" at Sud's Drive-Thru Liquor & Car Wash.

"So, how long has my *half*-brother been here?" she said. The "S" in "Sud's" blurred. She'd been on the verge of tears the entire day. It annoyed her.

"About five years." Jake offered Charlotte a menu.

"What's his name?"

"Adam. The fried mushrooms are decent. We could split an order."

"You're kidding." Charlotte shook her head. "Adam? That's really his name?"

"Yep. Why?"

"That's Chuck's middle name." The menu items ran together, a nonsensical jumble of letters. "What's Adam's last name?"

Jake didn't answer.

"It's Sutton, isn't it?"

"Yeah, sort of. His full name is Adam Sutton Mardian, but he dropped the Mardian about three years ago. I don't know why. If he changed his name legally or—"

"How old is he?"

"Fourteen."

"Holy shit. Of course. Of course, he is. That explains a hell of a lot."

"What do you mean?"

Charlotte stalled, putting the beer to her lips and wracking the rim against her teeth with a clink. The cool crispness hit the back of her throat. She could barely taste it.

"My parents split about 14 years ago." Charlotte plunked the beer back down on the bar. "Yeah. So, I was 14 when Chuck moved into the apartment above The Surly Sturgeon. It was the summer before my freshman year. I'm guessing Adam was the reason my parents got a divorce, and they just never told me."

"Oh, man, I shouldn't be in the middle of this." Jake raked fingers through his beard and tugged on the end. "I'm really, really sorry. Chuck never told me the whole story, just bits and pieces."

"Classic Chuck. Only tell them what they need to know, and make sure it doesn't make Chuck Sutton look bad."

Bea came shuffling over with silverware rolled in napkins. "Nice to see you back." Plopping the utensils down on the table, she plucked the menu from Charlotte's hand. "Ready, honey?"

Charlotte ordered, not much appreciating the side-eye she'd been getting from the marina owner since they walked in. No doubt, Bea had heard what transpired in Chuck's office. News traveled fast. The local gossip chain would be clinking for all its worth, and none of it would do her any favors, for sure. She waited until Bea was out of earshot and fired another question at her dinner partner.

"What about his mother? She knew Chuck pretty well, if she named her son after him. What's her story?"

"I don't really know," Jake said. "Her name is Sophia, but I've never met her. They aren't married. From what I can tell, I don't think Adam's mom has ever been back since dropping him off. I have no idea how they met."

"The kid said my name." Charlotte shrugged. "I heard him. He knew about me, even though I didn't know about him."

"Of course. Chuck talks about you all the time, Charlie."

"Please, don't call me that."

"Sorry. It's what your father—"

"I'm quite aware. Please, please, please don't call me Charlie."

"Message received, Charlotte. Got it."

"I hate nicknames." Charlotte looked through the nearest window at the nearly deserted boat slips. As was the custom, many owners pulled their boats out of the water just after Labor Day. The few remaining were likely owned by year-round residents or used commercially. Eventually, those, too, would be stored on land in anticipation of the lake freezing. Charlotte motioned to the *Erie Mermaid*, docked far out at the end of the pier, closest to open water. "Tell me about your business."

Jake took another swig from his bottle, placing the bottom back down precisely in its own water ring on the cardboard coaster. "I lease the *Mermaid* from a guy named Grant Warren. I've been chartering both a fishing boat and a sailboat for him for the past three years. Eventually, I hope to own my own charter business."

"Grant Warren? He was a year ahead of me. I thought he was a programmer or software engineer or something."

"He still is. Made millions on a software app for do-it-yourself house flippers." Jake took another sip of beer. "Now he consults for real estate companies out of Cleveland and Toledo."

"Grant lives around here?"

"Yep. He married the athletic director for Bay Area School District. Short, Asian, kind of fierce."

"Wait, what?" Charlotte laughed. "Is her name Jenny?"

"Yeah, *that's* it. I've only met her once."

"No way." Charlotte shook her head. "Grant Warren married Jenny Kim? Wow. I didn't think he had it in him. He had a huge crush on her in high school. It was so intense, he could barely speak when he was around her."

"Guess he got over his nerves." Jake motioned to Bea across the room. "Bea's Knees, can I get another?"

"Yeah, yeah, in a minute, Jakey." Bea threw her hands in the air, but winked before turning toward the beer taps.

"Bea's Knees? Jakey?" Charlotte arched a brow.

Jake shrugged. "Unlike you, I don't get too fussed about nicknames, particularly when given by someone who supplies me with free beer and a place to sleep."

"Fair." Charlotte laughed again, her heart lighter than it had been since she'd crossed over the Sandusky Bay. "I do like a free beer."

"You know, you should smile more. The fresh air is good for your teeth."

"Interesting phrase."

Jake's cheeks reddened. "My grandmother used to say that."

"I'm not judging."

"Pretty sure you are."

"Nah. Well, maybe a little, but it sounds to me like your grandmother gave good advice." Charlotte felt the sudden chill of cool air on the back of her neck. The door slammed back on its hinge, and a familiar voice echoed through the bar.

"Sorry I'm late, Bea. Trinity had an asthma attack. I had to walk Mom through giving her a breathing treatment again."

"Shit." Charlotte's hand instinctively flew to her nape, fingers closing over the ends of her pixie cut.

"No problem," Bea said. "Jake's awaitin' on a burger and fries, and there's a grilled chicken salad for Charlie Sutton. Remember her, honey? Same class as you, weren't she?"

Shit. Shit. Shit.

"Hey, Dana," Jake said. "How's it going?"

Charlotte winced. *I've died and gone straight to hell.* Dropping her shoulders, she slowly turned. Of course. Of course, Dana Fletcher. Mean girl. Most popular everything.

The redheaded nightmare from Charlotte's youth had dressed for both tips and comfort. Her breasts pushed against the thin cotton of a team shirt, and tight jeans hugged her gymnast's body. From Charlotte's roost, it didn't appear her nemesis had grown an inch since graduation, and hadn't even gained any weight. Dana was still Chihuahua size and just as cute as she'd been their senior year.

The bitch.

"Charlie?" Dana rushed to their table. "Oh, my gosh." Dana's delicate arms flew around Charlotte's neck, and her beautifully made-up cheek pressed against Charlotte's makeup-less one.

A faint whiff of lavender?

For real?

"You look amazing, Charlie."

Charlotte stared at the girl who called her The Tree all through high school. The girl who made fun of her clothes, her hair, her

50

height. The girl who drew a mustache on her during a church sleepover.

"When did you get here?" Dana said. "You live in Pittsburgh, right? Oh, my gosh, I read your articles all the time. So cool. I seriously might need your autograph."

"Um."

Dana.

The homecoming queen and prom queen and Ottawa County Fair queen and every other damn queen there ever was. She'd even gotten the boy—Charlotte's mini-crush, Mike McKenzie, star quarterback of the Bay Area Biting Walleyes football team.

"So cool that you've come home, Charlie."

Charlotte felt not one ounce of sorry to see the faintest of lines forming around Dana's lips and eyes. At least there was that.

"Charlie?" Dana said.

Jake nudged Charlotte with an elbow. "You okay?"

"Fine." Charlotte threw Jake a look and turned to Dana. "It's Charlotte, now, actually."

"Oh. Sure," Dana said. "Your dad always calls you Charlie. Sorry, I guess I've done the same in my head."

Better than The Tree, at least.

"I love your stories, especially the ones about growing up around here. Chuck always tells us when you've been published, so I've downloaded all the apps, *The Boston Globe*, *The New Yorker*. Great stuff. So impressive."

"Thanks." Charlotte twirled her fork, put it down, picked it up again. That her father had a clue she'd published a handful of essays came as almost as much of a surprise as Dana's compliments. "So, you stayed in the area?"

Dana nodded. "Sort of. I married Mike McKenzie right after graduation. He joined the Army, and we were stationed in Georgia, then moved back to raise our daughter in Marblehead. Trinity is five." Dana bowed her head and fiddled with the condiments.

"Where's he stationed now?" Charlotte wondered, with a whiff of hope, if they'd split. Had Dana not gone to college? Classic. No backup plan. Jump right into marrying your high school boyfriend and see what that gets you—a job slopping beer at The Surly Sturgeon.

Dana positioned catsup and mustard on either side of the salt and pepper. She slowly raised her gaze to meet Charlotte's. "Mike was killed two years ago, overseas. Mom's been helping me out ever since."

Charlotte sucked in a breath.

"At least I still have family around. And Jake. He's been known to babysit in a pinch." Dana threw Jake a hundred-watt smile, which he returned. "Trinity loves him."

Charlotte shook her head. "I'm so, so sorry."

"Yeah, me too." Dana shrugged.

"I can't even imagine how awful that must have been," Charlotte said. "Mike was a great guy."

"He sure was. We had a good life together, while it lasted."

"I bet."

Dana turned to go, paused, and then retraced her steps. The waitress's eyes stared into Charlotte's.

"We should do dinner sometime and catch up."

Charlotte's mouth dropped open. She shut it with a snap.

"I don't think—"

"Look, I'd understand if you didn't want to," Dana said. "You were always nice to everyone in school, Charlotte—nicer than most of us were to you, anyway. I'm sorry about that. I'm really sorry I didn't get to know you better back then. You have every reason to say 'no,' but think about it. I'd love to get together, if you're up for it."

Charlotte couldn't fathom how to process the invitation, let alone respond.

"Think about it." Dana shrugged again, the topic dead. "You and Sammy Macon still friends? Did you hear he took over the House of Beauty? Calls it The Clip Joint now."

"Classic. Chuck thought it was Clippers."

"Nope." Dana grinned. "It's definitely The Clip Joint. Caused a serious panic when the sign first went up. The locals were afraid he was opening a pot shop."

"Sammy and I haven't talked in a really long time."

"He's the best stylist in the area, for sure. You should let him know you're in town." Dana motioned to Charlotte's hair. "I always envied your short cut. So cute. Sammy's been trying to talk me into it for years, but I would never have the nerve to chop mine off like you did. Can I get you another beer?"

"Sure. Thanks."

Jake held his empty up to the light. "Me too, please."

"You bet. Your food should be out soon." Dana grabbed the empty bottle and turned, her denim-clad backside swish swishing its way across the room. Charlotte peeked at Jake under her lashes. *Swish.* He'd noticed, too. Hard not to. Dana was perfect.

Still freakin' perfect.

"I can't believe what happened to Mike. How horrible," Charlotte mumbled.

Jake nodded. "Yeah, Dana's had a rough time of it. She was a good friend of yours in high school?"

"Not exactly."

7

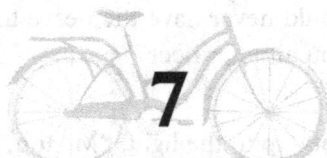

MIDDLE SCHOOL

"You hear? They're using The Tree as a coat rack during open house."

High-pitched giggles pushed against the back of Charlotte's bent head. She hunched her shoulders, sinking lower on the bench. She glanced at the clock above the cafeteria door—seven minutes and 32 seconds until fifth period.

"You hear? The Tree's got the personality of a 2x4."

"I don't get it."

"How stupid can you be?"

"I'm not stupid."

"A 2x4 is made from a tree, Stupid."

More laughter. Charlotte tucked herself further into the corner, concentrating on eating her re-hydrated mashed potatoes, mystery meat, and unnaturally green peas, which refused to stay on the fork. A little girl, age eight and missing since January, stared at her from a poster on the far cafeteria wall, her big eyes as stormy blue as the Biting Walleyes logo painted on the ceiling.

"You hear? The Tree's got a squirrel nut up her ass."

The last of the insults got the biggest response. Charlotte winced, recognizing Dana's voice. Kids at the adjoining table laughed. Some glanced at Charlotte, and their snickers faded. Among the popular girls, Dana was the cleverest at making the small people of the school feel even smaller or, in Charlotte's case, the tall people feel taller.

Unfortunately for The Tree, who had excellent hearing, ignoring the jokes was nearly impossible. Why did they always pick on her? She'd never done anything to them—had barely ever spoken to them. Charlotte tucked her chin to her chest. Tears spilled over and trickled into the collar of her sweatshirt. She pulled the hood and her thick hair forward to hide her face. She couldn't let them see her cry; it would only give them ammunition. With a sigh, she resumed picking at her mashed potatoes. She didn't want to care what they thought. She really didn't. But middle school was the beginning of her whole social career. When the area's small, individual school districts combined, merging the middle school students under one roof, she'd hoped she'd finally meet new people. Finally make friends. Instead, Charlotte found herself quite low on the Bay Area Biting Walleyes "popular" column. If she didn't turn things around... well, she didn't want to think about how many more years Dana and her bestie Nicki "The Hickey" Dinecky, and all the rest of the popular bitches, would make fun of her.

In front of *everybody.*

Everybody thought she was a loser. Charlotte glanced toward the adjoining table. Cute Bobby Myers looked her way and leaned over to whisper something in the ear of Teri Tory. Teri giggled and turned her back to Charlotte to talk to Katie "Pigtails" Wilson.

"Squirrel nuts. Get it?"

Everybody loved Dana. Everybody wanted to *be* her.

The social studies teacher, soft-hearted Miss Anderson, walked through the line of tables and stopped at the end of Charlotte's.

"Everything all right here?"

"Just fine, Miss Anderson," Dana said, her voice like honey.

"Charlotte?"

"Great." Jumping up from the table, Charlotte grabbed her nearly full tray and hurried across the room. She stared straight ahead at the blue-eyed girl on the poster. Why would the school put something like that up in the cafeteria? Were they trying to scare the students into not running away? Maybe the missing blue-eyed girl had the right idea. Maybe disappearing was the answer.

Charlotte felt the gaze of other students following her—hot pin-points prodding her from all angles as she passed. Dumping her leftovers in the trash, she bolted from the cafeteria to a stall in the girls' bathroom just across the hall.

* * * * *

That afternoon, Charlotte rolled over on her bed, tucking beneath her chin Yogi Bear-a, a threadbare teddy her father had given to her on her third birthday. A tissue, soggy and spent, lay on her pillow.

The day had only gotten worse. In the middle of Charlotte's sixth period math class, an announcement came over the loudspeaker.

Charlotte Sutton, please come to Principal Radcliff's office. Miss Sutton, come to the office immediately.

Everyone laughed except the new, cute kid, "Sammy from Miami," who sat right behind Charlotte. He seemed pretty chill and mouthed "give 'em hell" as she dragged her bookbag from the back of her chair.

Charlotte clutched Yogi Bear-a and wiped her damp cheek on his already soggy fur.

She had, most definitely, *not* given 'em hell. Not even close.

* * * * *

"Mr. Radcliff wants to see me?"

"Sit. Sit, Miss Sutton." The principal's secretary looked up from her desk. "Let's talk."

Like a good dog, Charlotte sank down onto a chair across from Ms. Levine's desk. "Tipsy" Levine, as most of the students called her behind her back, wasn't what Charlotte's mother considered a professional secretary. Elise called her a floozy. Tipsy's heart drummed, pitter-pat, beneath her black push-up bra under a sheer white blouse she'd paired with a cheap set of pearls, stiletto red pumps, and her too-short pencil skirt.

"Um, where's Mr. Radcliff?" Charlotte said.

"He's been called down to the math wing to proctor an algebra test, dear," Ms. Levine said. "I'm sure we can straighten this out, girl-to-girl. I'm here to help."

"Help?" Charlotte frowned. She wouldn't have minded talking with Mr. Radcliff. He wasn't very old, and he'd always been kind. He was an okay principal. On the other hand, Tipsy, who was about her parents' age, wasn't very good at her job. If the rumors were true, Tipsy would rather be assisting the football team.

But instead, she got me. The Tree.

"Now, what's this I hear about name-calling in the cafeteria? Miss Anderson seems to think you're at the center of it."

"I didn't do anything." Charlotte looked at her hands clasped so tightly in her lap that she could barely feel where one set of fingers ended and the other began.

"Hmmph. Ms. Anderson said as much. What happened, dear?"

"Nothing."

"Quite the contrary, it sounded like something. You'll not be returning to class until we get to the bottom of this."

Charlotte shifted in her seat. She hated Ms. Levine. She really, really hated her.

Without looking up, she mumbled the shortest of explanations. She left out the part about a squirrel nut up her ass. She didn't want to get suspended for cursing.

There was a brief silence. The toe of Charlotte's scuffed sneaker swirled a figure eight on the tile floor.

"Perhaps you could be a peer bully buddy mentor."

"What?" Charlotte pulled her head up.

"The district's new bullying program, dear." Ms. Levine smiled widely. She planted her elbows on her desk and her hands beneath her chin. In a high-pitched voice, the secretary explained the program and prattled on about friendships and spreading love and peace and harmony among the student body and being a leader among her peers.

Charlotte's mind numbed.

Peers. Peers. Peers.

"Peers listen to peers," Tipsy said. "You should be a mentor."

"Um... I'm the one being bullied, Ms. Levine," Charlotte said. "Could I get one of those mentors?"

"Peers listen to peers."

Not Charlotte's peers. Definitely *not* Charlotte's peers.

Damned squirrel nuts.

8

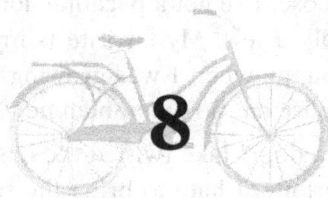

The Surly Sturgeon jukebox burst into life. Charlotte jumped, and the stool screeched and wobbled beneath her. Sydney stood and nudged her hand, giving her a reason to crouch down to the Aussie and wrap her arms around its neck. The tickle of dog hair on her cheek brought her a tiny bit of peace.

"You okay?" Jake said.

"Yeah, I'm good." Swiping her eyes, Charlotte returned to her chair and resumed picking at her salad. "Dana and I ran in completely different circles in high school. I'm actually really surprised she even remembers me."

"I get that. I've only kept up with a couple of college fraternity brothers and haven't talked to anyone from my hometown for years."

"Where'd you grow up?"

"Amish country, a couple of hours south of Cleveland. Unless you're a farmer, there are only so many options for jobs there. Nothing for a marine biologist, that's for sure. After I graduated, my parents sold the farm and moved to Florida. My brother is a computer programmer in California, so I'm on my own here, except for Sydney."

Charlotte looked down at the Aussie, lying now at Jake's feet with her chin on her paws.

"I'm pretty sure Sydney is awesome."

"Yep, and if you have treats, she'll be your best friend for life," Jake said.

"I've done a lot of pet-sitting since graduating." Charlotte peeled the label from her beer. "Writers don't make much money, unless you're Chuck, I suppose. I've got a part-time job in advertising, but I love dogs. Still walk a few. My favorite is my ex's lab, Alfredo. I always wanted a puppy when I was growing up, but my mother refused. Go figure. Elise has a Pomeranian now."

"I'll always have a dog." Jake twirled the base of his beer on its coaster. "Look, Charlotte, I hate to bring the subject back around to your dad, but—"

"I know what you're going to say. I should stay. It's the right thing to do. Chuck needs me. Whatever."

Jake shook his head. "I wasn't going to say any of that."

"But you'd think it." Charlotte sighed and turned to him. "I'm sorry... again. I seem to have to apologize to you too often."

"Maybe it's because you jump too quickly to your own conclusions." Jake smiled, but the edge to his voice hammered home the point. "Maybe?"

Charlotte shrugged. "Maybe. Look, I'm not disagreeing. I *know* it's the right thing to do, and I almost always do the right thing. That's the problem. I lose a piece of myself, bit by bit, each time I give in because of Chuck and his Chuck bullshit. He doesn't deserve my time because he never gave me his. Being back here sucks. Just. Plain. Sucks."

Jake allowed her rant to peter out on its own.

"And I don't really think he wants me here," Charlotte mumbled. "Not really."

"I see." Jake nodded. "All of this sounds a little... I don't know. I've never seen a selfish side to Chuck. Right now, he needs help, and you're the obvious one to help him. I get that the thing with your brother—"

"Half-brother."

"Half-brother. I get the thing with Adam is awkward, but your dad really wants you here. I'm sure of it. Maybe you should give him a chance."

Charlotte's finger traced the tip of her empty beer bottle, swirling at the speed of her thoughts. As always, the world revolved around Good-time Charlie, and he was calling all the shots. His many, little minions would defend him to the end.

Jake put his hand over hers. "Could you at least stay until after his neurology appointment on Monday? I went to his last one, and the doctor wants to speak to a family member. I don't want to put Adam through that, just yet."

The guilt was enough to bury her. She'd told the ad agency about her father's health, and they'd promised to be flexible, but she would not allow Chuck to be the reason she lost her job. She'd worked too hard.

"I'll try, but just until Monday afternoon. That's the best I can do."

*   *   *   *   *

It was full-on dark when Charlotte returned to the cottage, pulled the rocker back out of her car, and gently placed it on the front porch; she'd rather no one asked why it had traveled from upstairs to down. Through the thin curtains on the lower level, she spied her father in his leather recliner watching television. Adam stood at the kitchen counter.

Her dad thrust his fist in the air and gave a loud whoop. His son rushed to join him, the two identical in their shared excitement. They were focused on a college football game.

Charlotte felt a mix of emotions as she observed their exchange. She never had that. Could never have that. And there was absolutely nothing she could do to change those circumstances.

She went around back and retrieved her suitcase from her car. When she entered the kitchen, a waft of garlic hit her. Bread sat on the cutting board, a pan of red sauce bubbled on the stove, and a large vat of pasta boiled, sending steam into the air. Charlotte shut the door behind her. There was a pause in the voices from the living room, and Adam walked back into the kitchen and gave Charlotte a careful nod.

"Hello. It smells really good in here," Charlotte said. "Did you do all this?"

"Yeah. Dad wasn't up to cooking dinner, and I got hungry." The teen turned his back to her, retrieved the cutting board, and grabbed a knife from the block on the counter. He went quiet, carving away at the bread loaf with quick, even strokes.

"We haven't been introduced. I'm Charlotte."

He stopped cutting and looked down at the loaf in his hand.

"Yeah. I'm Adam." He shrugged, and the scrape of the knife returned, slicing the awkward silence. His stroke was not so even now.

"Well, it sure smells good." Charlotte stared at the boy's back, wondering what he thought of all this. "I shouldn't have eaten at the bar."

Adam's shoulders hunched. Maybe waiting and wondering how he could escape the conversation? Charlotte wasn't the only one with a new sibling, and as pissed as she was for not knowing Adam existed, it wasn't the kid's fault their dad had pulled a Chuck. Giving her half-brother back his kitchen, she took a steadying breath and inched toward the living room. She paused in the doorway.

"Hey, Chuck. What's playing?"

"OSU versus Michigan and some highlights from last weekend's Cleveland-Pittsburgh game." Chuck's attention did not stray from the television. "A tie with Pittsburgh is a win, in my book."

Charlotte set her suitcase by the stairs.

I stayed. Do you even care?

Her father continued to watch the game, the emotional reunion of just a few hours before seemingly already forgotten.

Charlotte veered to the bookshelf in the corner, and she trailed her fingers over the well-worn paperbacks. Chuck's collection had a little bit of everything, including a lot of sports biographies and, of course, the classics. On the bottom shelf, she spied several copies of her father's own *Smokin' Smokey Joe*, his bestselling biography about Smoky Joe Wood, an early 1900s pitcher and outfielder. Did Chuck keep the convenient stash handy for when the stray fan came a-knocking?

"Chuck Sutton," he'd say, thrusting out his hand. *"How would you like me to sign it? Love, Chuck? Plenty more homeruns where that came from."*

"Do they have a shot at a winning season this year?" she said.

"What?"

She ran trembling fingers over the bookshelf titles and glanced over her shoulder. "Cleveland. Think they could have a winning season?"

"Oh. Nah. Probably not. That's just dreamin', Charlie."

Charlotte frowned. At least he recognized her. Her chest tight, she leaned against the nearby wall. The small talk would surely kill her; she shouldn't have come.

"So, I... I guess I'll call my boss and tell her I plan to stay for your neurology appointment. It's Monday, right?"

Chuck pulled his gaze from the television. "What?"

"Your neurology appointment? When is it?"

"Monday. Ten o'clock," Adam said, appearing by her side. He thrust a calendar into her hands. "The office is in Marblehead."

"Thanks." Glancing at her father, Charlotte pulled her phone from her pocket and took a picture of the entire month of November. Adam disappeared back into the kitchen. He was obviously taking on more responsibility and emotional crap than an average 14-year-old should ever have to deal with.

And Chuck? Completely clueless.

Charlotte returned to the kitchen and laid the calendar on the corner of the countertop. "Thanks for keeping track of things."

"He has a calendar on his cell, too." Adam motioned to a phone resting in the tray on the windowsill, next to the hook holding a set of car keys. "Passcode to his phone is 6789, and his email is 'Charlieanne'."

"I'm sorry?"

"Char-lie-anne," Adam repeated, his voice clipped. "Anne with an 'e'." He grabbed the phone and smoothly tossed it toward Charlotte. She barely caught the device mid-air, bumbling it nearly as badly as the many balls she'd let slip through her fingers over the years.

"Oh." The weight of Chuck's phone felt like lead in Charlotte's hand. Adam turned away, and she touched the screen. A picture of her brother wearing a baseball uniform and holding a trophy popped into view as the screensaver. Charlotte turned the phone over and hurried across the kitchen to place it back on its tray, screen side down.

Why would Chuck use her name as a passcode? Why not "Adam" or "Lakeside" or "newspaper" or even "Smokey Joe?" Anything, anything at all but "Charlieanne?" Her father didn't deserve to use her name as a passcode. It was *her* name. She could use it, but he could not. He'd never earned that right.

* * * * *

Charlotte sat at the table nibbling a corner of a piece of garlic bread and pushing a mound of sauce-soaked noodles across her plate. After dinner, Adam disappeared upstairs. She could hear him clattering about. The exposed ceiling above her head still showed open beams; no insulation, not even carpet, existed between the floors, allowing every little sound to reverberate throughout the house.

Her father hunkered down in his recliner. Charlotte went to the kitchen to take care of the dishes. In Lakeside, "modern" had always been a four-letter word. They were fortunate to have a garbage disposal, but a dishwasher had never been in the cards. Dumping the leftovers into plastic containers, she plunked the dirty dishes in the sink and filled it with soapy water. She barely registered the dark shadow of a squirrel climbing the tree just outside the kitchen window. As a child, before the early growth spurt had her shooting up past the top of her petite mother's head, Charlotte had stood on a stool to dry, while her mother washed. Charlotte glanced back through the door to where her father sat in his recliner, exactly where he always sat while she and her mother cleaned up. Charlotte refocused on the matter at hand, not minding the sting of the too-hot water. Washing dishes gave her time to think. Time to justify her intent to leave Lakeside again, as quickly as possible.

She dried the dishes, put them away, and trudged back into the living room. As she grabbed a copy of her father's *Smokin' Smokey Joe* from the bookshelf, the book next to the biography slid out onto the floor. Charlotte reached to put it back and paused. The leather-bound journal looked suspiciously like one of the many she'd filled as a teenager. She opened the cover. In her father's messy scrawl, the word "Charlie" had been written in the bottom right corner of the otherwise blank first page.

Oh, God. He didn't.

She fanned the pages, expecting her own journal entries in her own rounded swoops and swirls, but, instead, her father's spidery handwriting swept past. She paused at an early page with a date and the heading "Charlotte, age six."

> *It's a snowy day in December, the white caps forming over the dock like a layer of frosted icing. From the window, I watched my little girl all bundled up to her eyebrows in purple, like usual, out beneath the cottonwoods. For hours, she rolled snow into a ball, back and forth, leaving a trail of darkened grass.*
>
> *She's a determined little thing, my Charlie. All it takes is all you've got, I always say. Well, it took her a few tries, but she managed to pull the middle section of the snowman up onto the base all by herself. I finished my article just in time to run out and offer to lift up the head, but she wanted to do it. Insisted on doing it. She held the head, and I lifted*

*her up instead, so she could finish the job. Elise gave her one
of my old scarves and a baseball hat, a carrot for the nose,
and a bag of red licorice sticks to use for the mouth. We found
a couple of barren twigs for the arms and even sacrificed
one of my old, wooden bats. Charlie called the snowman
"Snow-Daddy." I sure got a chuckle out of that.*

Charlotte snapped the cover closed and rammed the journal
back on the shelf. She could feel the heat in her cheeks, like the time
Elise had been out shopping and Charlotte accidentally stumbled
upon her mother's stash of explicit magazines—three well-worn
copies hidden in her sweater drawer. Only about 11 years old, at
the time, Charlotte remembered flipping through them and getting
a real eyeful. Chuck's journal disturbed her far more than the nude
male photos had.

Her heart beating fast, she made her way to the end of the couch
and sat down as far away from her father as possible. Adam tromped
back down the stairs. He was dressed all in black, with a leather
jacket draped over his arm and a drawstring bag hanging from his
shoulder.

"Headin' out, Dad."

Chuck focused on Adam in a blink. "Not tonight, son."

Charlotte glanced at her phone. It was nearly ten o'clock on a
Saturday—getting-in-trouble-with-friends time. She couldn't count
the number of Saturdays she'd spent driving all over Marblehead
Peninsula looking for entertainment with Sammy. Most of it had
been innocent enough. Some of it not so much.

"But, Dad—"

"No, 'but, Dad.' Did you finish your English paper?"

"Seriously? You know I did. Come on. You proofed it. It was due
yesterday. I already turned it in."

"Right. Sorry," Chuck said. "I don't want you going out tonight."

"Ah, man. It's a Saturday. I told Shen I'd be over after dinner.
What's the big deal?"

Chuck's eyes closed. "Your sister is here. That's the big deal."

Oh. No. He. Didn't.

Charlotte bit back the buzz of anger again racing to the surface. From the look on Adam's face, he wasn't any happier.

Chuck had never bothered to be a father to her—not really. When it came to an argument, he never yelled like Elise, but always had more verbal ammunition. Here he was, using a heavier hand with Adam and throwing her into the middle of it, as some sort of bribe-like threat.

"Come watch the replays with us," added Chuck. "That's what a good son would do."

"Charlotte can watch with you." Adam shot her a look, a red stain painting his cheeks. "You don't need me."

Charlotte flinched. "Adam, I don't—"

"That's why you're here, right, to take control? To be his babysitter?"

"I'm no babysitter."

Adam laughed, the sound a hollow crack. "Yeah, right. Dad might need one, but I sure as hell don't. I'm going out."

Charlotte stood. "Forget it. Forget the whole damned thing. It's been a really long day. I'm going to bed. You two can work out... whatever this is." Her hand wavered in the air between them like a drunken bird. She wanted nothing more than to remove herself from her recently discovered, smart-mouthed half-brother. And her father. And the babysitting responsibility of either or both of them.

"That was unnecessary," Chuck said. "Both of you should be ashamed of yourselves."

Ignoring her father, Charlotte grabbed her suitcase and bounded upstairs, straight to the guest bedroom at the farthest end of the second-floor hallway. She pressed her forehead against the frame of the door and waited for her anger to subside. The sudden slam of the front door below sent a vibration through the wood.

Adam had apparently won the battle.

It was hard to tell just how far her father's disease may have progressed. Would he remember the fight an hour from now or that his son was out on a Saturday night, doing whatever?

Pushing the door open, Charlotte stepped into the bedroom.

"No way." Her gaze flitted from one corner to the other and back again.

Charlotte's childish past—the white twin bed with the wrought-iron frame, a threadbare lavender chenille bedspread, her stuffed teddy Yogi Bear-a, and the white-painted cedar chest with the honey stain peeking through on the worn corners—filled the room. The walls had been painted the exact same shade of pale purple as her childhood room—now Adam's.

Near the window sat the Victorian dollhouse she'd played with endlessly as a child. She'd made up stories about the inhabitants, a picket-fence-like family of five—Mommy, Daddy, Girl, Baby Brother, and the family pet, Dog. Girl was Charlotte, of course. She couldn't remember what she had last called Baby Brother, whom she'd wanted in real life for the longest time but never gotten.

Until now.

The name had changed frequently. Regardless, it had absolutely *never* been Adam Sutton Mardian.

Charlotte picked up the collie dog figurine and moved it to the end of a bed where Girl was tucked in for the night. Charlotte re-arranged the living room to accommodate Mommy at the kitchen sink and Daddy on the sofa watching television. A football replay, no doubt. She placed Baby Brother in the attic room, with the crib and a blanket no bigger than a postage stamp. They all needed their rest. It was true. It had been a very, very long day. A long, stressful, anxiety-filled, crappy-assed day.

* * * * *

Charlotte heard Chuck turn off the television about an hour after she went to bed. The sounds of the house were no longer as familiar to her. The winds whipped, setting a tree limb snapping against her window. From her bed, she saw the waterfront path, faintly outlined by the dim, yellow haze of sporadically placed light poles. Everything was the same but different.

Her eyes itched with exhaustion and unspent tears. She kept looking out at the black of the lake, viewed at a different angle than she'd grown up with seemingly a thousand years before. Her mind wouldn't shut off. Spinning, spinning.

What was her brother's real story? She deserved an explanation. The spotty outline Jake had provided had too many holes. Her father had never really been much of a father—to her, at least. Had Adam fared better?

Doubtful.

It was almost two in the morning when the Rusty Banana swerved down the footpath from the direction of the pavilion, breaking every Lakeside rule prohibiting bikes in the park. Charlotte's lips twitched at the memory of her own teenage flaunting of authority. The figure in black slowed in front of Sutton's Choice and cycled out of sight. A few moments later, there was the faint click of the backdoor opening and shutting.

Adam was home. With a huff of breath, Charlotte rolled over and burrowed further into the folds of chenille. Finally, her eyelids drooped, fluttered.

Her brother miscalculated the squeaky staircase on his way up to bed. Charlotte sighed and rolled over with her last conscious thought.

Amateur.

She quickly drifted into slumber.

9

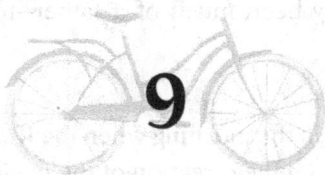

Charlotte startled awake and shot up to a seated position, her heart racing. Fragmented dreams fell into place like a puzzle. She'd run through the cottage, opening every door and looking for something. Someone. The last place she'd searched was her old bedroom, and she'd stumbled out onto the porch, where a strange woman with long, dark hair sat feeding a baby in her mother's rocker. She sang in a husky voice dripping with sorrow. The dream had seemed so real. The wind whistled through the trees, and the mist coming off the water dampened her fingers as she reached out to touch the child.

To touch Adam.

She groaned and reached for her phone. Almost nine o'clock—well past her usual waking hour, even on a Sunday. She closed her eyes, but the faint voices of talking heads from below nudged her. Chuck was awake and watching television.

It didn't matter that it was a new day. Nothing had changed. She was no closer to the answers she sought. No closer to understanding.

How could she have a brother? How could he not tell her?

Eyes puffy and head thumping, Charlotte gave up the fight and crept from her bed. She dragged on clothes and went downstairs.

"That's what I'm talking about," Chuck said, raising his fist in the air. He sat in his usual chair watching what appeared to be the news highlights of the expected Sunday football matchups. He glanced away from the television and smiled.

"Ah. Good morning, Charlie. It's a beautiful day for football."

"If you say so."

"Coffee is already brewed," Chuck said. "Sounds like you could use a cup."

"Sure." Charlotte trudged into the kitchen and fetched a mug. How could he be so positively oblivious? It was a mistake to come.

She shuddered, feeling a chill cross her shoulder blades. She wrapped her hands around the hot beverage and exited the kitchen. Like a magnet resisting its opposite, she forced herself toward the couch. She inched down onto the edge of the cushions.

"You sleep okay, kid?"

Charlotte shrugged. On the floor at her feet sat a basket of fresh laundry, not yet folded, the fabrics a tangle of blue, brown, gray, and black.

"If I'd have known you were coming, I would have gotten a new mattress for your bed," Chuck said. "Pretty sure that lumpy thing you've got is older than you are."

Charlotte stared at the laundry. She should have gotten more sleep. She wasn't equipped to deal with his nonsense. She simply wasn't. She raised the coffee to her lips, barely registering the sting of the scalding brew, and set it on the side table.

Why *had* she returned? Was she expecting a first-place ribbon? A gold star? Was that it? Duty had called her home, but what was the point? Her father didn't need her; he had Adam.

She shouldn't care.

I don't. I don't care at all.

"You okay? You look tired, Charlie."

She pressed her chin to her chest and took a deep breath. The blues and browns and grays swam before her eyes.

Chuck cleared his throat. "Real tired."

"Of course, I'm tired. I'm tired as shit." The expletive, like water from a dam, burst from Charlotte with giddy relief. She raised her head. "I only got a few hours of sleep."

Chuck leaned over and patted Charlotte's hand, clenching the couch arm.

"We'll get you a new mattress. Take you right up to Sandusky to Mattress Mania and pick out something—"

"I don't need a damned mattress."

Charlotte's shoulders shook. She was done. Done tiptoeing around the questions she had. Done making excuses for her father and tossing on her lumpy, old mattress for hours in the night.

Done.

"Okay," Chuck said. "What do you—"

"Please, just stop." Charlotte faced her father. "How can you be like this? How can you sit there and ramble on about mattresses and act like everything is perfectly normal after yesterday?"

"I don't—"

"I have a brother you never told me about. You can't just act like Adam dropped from the sky and has always been here. I don't know him. I don't know anything about him. What the hell?"

"Charlie, I—"

"You weren't ever going to tell me, were you? *Were* you? Don't you think I deserve to know what happened? So, help me. If you won't explain, I'll leave. Right. Damn. Now."

"Charlie—"

"Tell me."

A weight lifted from her chest with the demand. She had never demanded anything of her father before. She had never demanded anything of anyone. Ever.

The talking heads in the background droned. Chuck pressed a button on the clicker, and the television went silent. Placing the

72

device on the end table, he folded his hands in his lap. Time stretched as he stared at the blank screen.

Was he intentionally ignoring her?

"Chuck?"

Charlotte's father looked down, then picked a lint fluff from his shirt and examined it, like it was the most interesting object in the world.

"For real? You've seriously got to be kidding me." Charlotte bolted for the stairs. "I'm out."

"Do you really want to have this conversation, kid? I'd rather you didn't."

Charlotte's steps stalled. She turned.

Chuck's body was still. Calm. But his hands were planted on the arms of the chair, gripping hard enough to make an indent.

"It's easier to walk away," Chuck said. "We both know that's what I'd do."

"I don't—"

"This will only make things worse. Much, much worse. You won't like what I have to say, Charlie. I can guarantee it. So, I'm asking—do you *really* want to have this conversation? Are you quite sure?"

Chuck's face showed no emotion.

"What kind of question is that?" Charlotte's voice came out as a croak. She reached behind her, seeking the support of the bead-board wall. "Of course, I'm sure."

"Once it's out there, I can't put it back."

Chuck's voice was so soft, Charlotte could barely hear his words.

"I can't change it, Charlie," Chuck whispered. "I can't. Even if I wanted to."

"Maybe you should have thought about that before you cheated on Mom."

Charlotte's father shook his head. "I don't want—"

"I don't really care what you want." Charlotte crossed her arms. "I need to know. You owe me this. Be a grown-ass adult and take some responsibility."

Chuck studied her for a moment then nodded. "Very well." He motioned to the couch. "Please, sit down. Let's at least be civilized about it."

"Fine." Charlotte retraced her steps and sank onto the cushions. Wanting something to do with her hands, she tossed the load of laundry upside down on the sofa, forming a mounded barrier between them. She plucked a towel from the pile, her fingers stiff as she quickly folded it into a sloppy, irritable square.

"Well?" Charlotte glanced at her father.

Chuck sighed. "You were a bit younger than Adam is now when it happened. It was a woman I met at a stadium."

Charlotte sucked in a breath. Anger rose again and threatened to choke her. Adam's story summed up in just a handful of words.

It was that simple. Just what I expected.

She'd hoped it would be a less seedy story, but no. Her fingers twisted the towel, but she couldn't feel the fabric. It was as if she were numb.

"So, basically, you hooked up with the first willing fan that came along."

"No. I didn't... *hook up* with a fan. Willing or otherwise. What type of person do you take me for?"

Charlotte's jaw clenched, the need to control her reaction a physical pain. "The type of person who would cheat on his wife. The self-absorbed type of person who would raise his son without telling his daughter she had a brother. That type of person."

Chuck winced. "I guess I kind of deserve that."

"You think?" Charlotte returned her attention to the laundry, trying to keep her tongue in check, a nearly impossible task. Questions filled her head, and the room fell silent again.

Chuck cleared his throat. "Perhaps, we should try this some other—"

"No."

She wouldn't let him back out, but she also wouldn't get any answers if she pushed him too hard. Regardless, she'd be lucky to get even *half* the story, and, for sure, none of it would be her father's fault. But half was more than none. A lot more.

"Please. Go on."

"Right." Chuck paused. "Sophia Mardian was a sports therapist working with a national baseball team. For one of the networks, I interviewed her for a story I was doing on steroid use."

"Sounds like the story wasn't the only thing you were doing."

Chuck frowned. "If you're going to be crass, we can put this topic to bed right now."

Charlotte felt exactly that. *Crass. Rude. Ugly.*

Deflated, like a day-old balloon.

Charlotte shrugged. "I didn't mean—"

"Adam's mother was a good person," Chuck said. "Not some pick-up, for Christ's sake."

"I don't care how good she was. You were married. It doesn't excuse it. Not by a mile."

"No, it doesn't, but I don't know how better to explain this to you. Your mom and I weren't meant to stay together, kid. I loved her, but she was always so mad about—"

"Stop!" Charlotte leaned forward and jabbed a finger in the air, an arrow aimed for her father's head. "Don't you blame Mom for this. She had a reason to be mad. Lots of reasons."

"I'm sorry. I didn't mean for it to come out like that, but you've got to understand. Elise was always finding fault. I could never please her."

"You hardly tried. At least *she* was around. *You* were *never* around."

"You are absolutely right." Chuck shook his head. "It was easier that way for all of us, Charlie. Trust me. I'm not trying to lay the blame on your mother. There's plenty of blame to share, but Elise and I were like oil and water. When I met Sophia, it was very different."

"Bullshit." Charlotte dropped a Bay Area sweatshirt into the basket, sending it back into crumpled disarray.

"I'm just trying to explain."

"By throwing shade on Mom."

"I suppose you would see it that way." Chuck sighed. "You always took your mother's side, and I never gave you a reason not to."

"I shouldn't have to take a side. Quit talking about what Mom did and start talking about what *you* did."

Chuck's face paled. "I'm sorry. Really, I am."

"Are you going to tell me about Adam, or not?"

"Right. Sorry. When my book received an award, Sophia emailed and asked to meet, so I could autograph her copy." Chuck's focus faded to a different time and place. "I was flattered, and I agreed."

"Sex. Fan."

"It wasn't like that." Chuck pushed himself to the edge of his seat, his gaze boring into Charlotte's. "We just met for coffee."

"And she made you feel what? Important? Validated?"

"Yes, actually. Validated is a very good word for it. Your mother and I were long past validating each other. I couldn't even wear the right shirt to dinner."

The words wormed their way into Charlotte's head, planting a tiny seed of doubt. Chuck and Elise had always fought, but Charlotte never listened closely to their bickering, never really tore it apart and analyzed it to get to the heart of the argument. But subconsciously, she thought she understood. She had not told Elise about Chuck's health and the unexpected trip to Ohio for a reason. The mention of him usually brought out her mother's screechy, judgmental side. In short, she'd have a shit fit.

Chuck was right; Charlotte had always, naturally, sided with her mother. But why not? Elise had been a bit excessive at times, but a good parent. She'd come to every game. She'd baked cookies for class parties. She'd served as PTA President and volunteered whenever asked. She'd taken Charlotte shopping and to the movies and for haircuts and doctors' appointments.

Elise had always been there. Chuck had not.

"Your mom and I were just a couple of dumb kids when we got married," Chuck said. "Hell, she was only 22—six years younger than you are now. I was a couple of years older and had just gotten called up to the big leagues. We were high on life. We loved each other, but we were both too young to realize we weren't right for each other. Back then, everybody got married early. I'm not blaming your mom, Charlie. Really. But if we hadn't had you a few years later, we might not have stayed married nearly as long as we did."

"What? You didn't want children either? You didn't even *want* me?" Charlotte couldn't hide the hatred in her words. "I guess you really screwed that up, didn't you, Chuck? Twice even."

"I didn't mean—"

"Forget it." Charlotte stood.

"Please, sit down, Charlie. You wanted to know everything. Well, here's everything."

Eff you, Chuck. And your everything.

Dread weighed on her shoulders, pushing Charlotte back into her seat. She *had* asked for it.

"Look, Elise was a real pistol." Chuck swept a hand over his brow. "Still is. I loved her for it, but she made me feel a little small sometimes, is all. We were always fighting about something or other. Elise always won, and I always let her. It was much easier that way."

Charlotte gritted her teeth. "Tell. Me. About. Adam."

"Right." Chuck nodded. "Sophia and I met for drinks whenever I was in Cleveland. She was a huge baseball nut. We'd end up at a sports bar, taking in a game and talking about anything. Everything." Chuck smiled. "I liked her. I liked her a lot, actually. Anyway, we were nothing but two friends with the same interest in sports and a reason to share a meal. We met like that, for years. We were just friends."

"Until you weren't."

"I didn't plan for it to happen, kid. Your mother and I had a fight. Worse than usual. I was upset and feeling sorry for myself. Sophia listened. We both drank way too much that night, and one thing led to another. We ended up back at my hotel."

Chuck put his hand to his face again, rubbing his temples. "It was a one-time thing. Neither of us felt right about it, and we agreed to never see each other again. The guilt ate me up, and I finally told your mother everything. That's when it all really came to a head. We gave it nearly a year and tried to make it work for your sake. But by that point, neither of us wanted to stay in the marriage. My indiscretion was an excuse to end it."

Charlotte remembered the divorce. The months leading up to her fourteenth birthday—and her parents' final split just a couple of weeks after—had been the hardest time of her life. She'd thought, deep down, it was somehow her fault.

"That's that. It happened," Chuck said, "and if it hadn't been Sophia, it would have likely been someone else."

Charlotte shook her head. "You don't even sound sorry."

"I will never regret it, if that's what you're asking."

"How could you say that?" Charlotte snapped. "You don't regret the divorce? You don't regret cheating on Mom?"

"Of course, I regret *that*." Chuck leaned forward in his chair, again, his gaze pinning her to the cushions. "Believe me. I never meant to hurt either of you, but I don't regret being Adam's father. Having him. I love my son. I might not deserve what I've been given, but he's one of the best gifts I've ever received. I have Sophia to thank for that."

Charlotte rose and walked to the north windows. The wind sent the tree limbs above the front porch into a furious hula. The morning sun glimmered on the lake, as the water swept up onto the rocks, cresting in curls of angry, white foam. Charlotte acknowledged the irony. She and the lake shared the same mood. It was an angry day. A restless day.

Chuck had every right to love his son. Though she despised him for his adultery, his actions weren't really what angered Charlotte most. It was that someone outside their family mattered more to him than she and her mother had, or likely ever would. It boiled down to that, if she looked at it from every angle. Chuck preferred spending time with Sophia for years, being away from Lakeside whenever possible, while Charlotte tried and failed, miserably, at every sport known to man—not for herself but for him.

And cheating on their family resulted in a son who excelled at sports.

That's messed up. Really messed up.

"Exactly when did Adam come here?" Charlotte asked, though Jake had told her the gist.

"Five years ago. He was nine, Charlie. You didn't know about him, but neither did I until his mom showed up on my doorstep one day with a surprise."

"Hell of a surprise."

"Yes. Yes, he certainly was."

"Why did she bring him here? Where is she?"

Chuck considered Charlotte, as if deciding how much he should reveal.

"What happened, Chuck?"

"Sophia became addicted to prescription meds after a surgery." The pain in Chuck's eyes said more than the words. "She wanted a better life for our son while she got herself clean. Unfortunately, rehab didn't work. She's in prison now for drug-related offenses."

"Oh, my god. What did she do?"

"Aggravated vehicular homicide," Chuck said. "She was high on painkillers when her vehicle went off the road and hit a tree. Adam wasn't in the car, but a college kid she was mentoring was. He was killed on contact."

"She... killed someone?" Bile rose in Charlotte's throat. How could something like this happen?

"It was an accident, but yes."

"That's horrible. Why in the hell didn't you tell me?"

"I tried. Sort of." Chuck dipped his chin. "I called you a few times, but you never picked up. How do you tell your daughter that kind of news? How could I just leave a message about Adam? I didn't know what to say. I didn't know how to explain any of it."

My god.

Charlotte's mind churned at warp speed. Her gaze darted to the stairs to the second floor. Could her brother hear them through the thin cottage walls?

"Is Adam awake?"

"He's not here," Chuck said. "Left about an hour ago to play basketball with his friends, I think. Course, no telling if I'm remembering right, to be truthful."

"Does he know about his mom?"

"Yes. I used to take him to visit Sophia once a month. Things changed after she was arrested. About three years ago, she turned us away. Embarrassed, I suppose. We were told she didn't want us to return."

"That's awful."

"Adam hasn't seen or talked to his mother since, though I keep trying. I petitioned to take full custody. He's my son, and I want to do right by him."

"I wasn't questioning his paternity," Charlotte said. "All you have to do is look at him to know he's yours."

"The same can be said of you, Charlie."

Charlotte shook her head. She had asked for the truth, but the truth was too much.

Too much anger.

Too much loss.

Too much hurt.

Adam ended up in Lakeside through no fault of his own—just a messed-up kid, as she'd been, with teen angst and dumb-assed parents. But on a much more dramatic scale. It was crazy. Her father had missed most of her growing-up years, but, with Adam, he hadn't even been given a choice. Maybe it was Chuck's punishment for being absent in her own life, but Adam had been punished by her father's absence, too, and had not deserved what he was dealt.

"Does Mom know?"

Chuck dipped his head, his voice barely audible. "I told her when Adam moved in."

"You've got to be kidding me. What the hell?"

"She said I needed to be the one to explain this to you, Charlie. She knew you'd be upset. Your mother and I agreed on that, at least."

Charlotte thought back to age 14. To the divorce. To being bullied by her peers.

Getting upset, for any number of reasons, had been a weekly thing, sometimes daily, but really, in comparison to Adam's situation, it could have been far worse.

"Is he all right? Doing okay in school?" she said. "I mean, it's a lot to deal with."

"He's not a straight-A student like you were, but he does just fine." Chuck smiled for the first time that morning, his pride a palpable thing. "He keeps his grades up enough to stay on the baseball team and basketball team. Your brother has handled everything remarkably well, all things considered. I think he struggles, at times, to find his place in this community, though. He's not been a Lakesider for very long, of course, and that makes it a little difficult."

A groan escaped Charlotte's lips. "You don't need to tell me. I didn't exactly fit in either. Some people can be vicious."

Chuck studied his daughter for a moment. "And some people— some *Lakesiders*—are the most generous you'll ever meet. You'll have your good and your bad, no matter where you live. Lakeside isn't any different than any other small town, Charlie. Not really any different than a big city, either. Lumping everyone into the same pot is like saying canned chili is the same thing as your mother's homemade broccoli cheddar soup."

"Sure, Chuck, but middle school and high school sucked. No question."

"If being a teenager was easy, we'd never have a reason to grow up."

"If you say so."

"I do. Besides," Chuck said, "I thought *I* was the reason you left."

Charlotte nodded. "Not wrong. Living under your shadow wasn't much fun, either."

"Well, that shouldn't be a problem now." Chuck shrugged. "I'm just a washed-up old reporter who can't remember which advertisers paid for which issues. Give me a few more months, and we won't have any advertisers left to worry about, let alone a family newspaper."

"The guilt trip won't work." Charlotte pushed the laundry aside. "When does Adam's mom get out of prison?"

Chuck shook his head. "Not anytime soon. He's with me until he heads to college. That's what worries me. Sophia has no family. If the Alzheimer's progresses the way my doctor thinks it will, I may not be well enough to raise Adam. It's not likely, but he could even be taken from me if no one steps up. Until he turns 18, there is that risk."

"Wait, what? I don't understand."

Chuck nodded. "Worst case, if I become mentally incompetent, Adam could be put under the government's care. I can't risk that. I have to plan ahead."

"He's your son. They can't just take him away."

"It's not likely, but someone has to be here, Charlie, if I'm not able to be a parent to him. At the very least, I need to assign a preferred guardian. A Power of Attorney would take care of my health care wishes, my finances, and when I—"

"Don't be so dramatic, Chuck." Charlotte rolled her head, loosening the knots in her neck. "You're still... competent."

"For how long? There's no telling when I won't be. Adam needs stability. I may not be able to give him that much longer."

Charlotte stared down at the Bay Area Biting Walleyes t-shirt in her lap. Her nerves tightened like a high wire—the soft, cotton fabric in her hands sandpaper to the touch.

"You're my next of kin." Chuck scratched a patch of whiskers, the rasp of nails on skin.

"I know it's asking a lot, but I've got the legal paperwork all ready to go and—"

This was the set-up?

"You're crazy," Charlotte whispered. "Completely crazy." Her head swiveled back and forth. "How could you ask that of me? We haven't spoken in 10 years."

"I'm sorry."

"I'm sorry? It's not that damn simple. Since graduation, you haven't communicated with me." Charlotte rose with her voice. She stood over her father and allowed the hurt to billow out of her like vomit. "You didn't call. You didn't even write a letter, and now you want me to take responsibility for you?" Charlotte's gaze met her father's, then skittered away. "*And* the brother I didn't know I had?"

"Oh, now, Charlie—"

"Quit calling me that. I hate that name. I've *always* hated that name."

"I'm sorry, kid. I didn't mean—"

"I'm not a kid, either."

"You are to me. You'll always be *my* kid."

"Just not the son you always wanted, huh, Chuck?"

"How could you ever think—"

"I can't stay. I'll go to your doctor's appointment tomorrow, but you'll have to figure out something from there. I've got to go back to Pittsburgh." Charlotte swept up the folded laundry and plunked it in the basket. "I've got a job. I can't stay, Chuck; I won't."

Chuck pulled in a breath, his spine straight, his eyes glued to unseen images across the room.

"But thank you for finally telling me Adam's story."

Charlotte ran from the room.

10

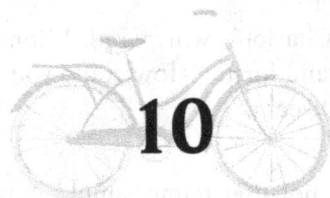

Charlotte grabbed her coat and keys. She'd go for a drive around the peninsula. Escape Sutton's Choice.

The air was crisp, the sun shining, as she turned onto Second Street and headed through town. Driving slowly, she allowed the quiet streets, mostly deserted in the off-season, to calm her racing heart. Along the sidewalks fronting the businesses, someone had decorated each corner with cornstalks and mums. A feral, black cat darted from beside The Patio Restaurant, a favorite donut haunt, to cross the road. Charlotte slowed and swerved around the creature.

It was all so impossible to comprehend. Chuck's story helped her understand Adam's history—what led to her even having a half-brother—but it hadn't helped her reconcile her own feelings about her father. Not really. As he'd warned, she hadn't liked what he had to say.

Taking a side street, she crept past the Hoover Auditorium, a long, brick structure hunched on an entire block of its own. Elise had taken her to see entertainment there most summer evenings from the time she was very young. Those had been good nights, with or without Chuck, but on the rare occasion they were all together as a family, the performance of the singer or orchestra or comedian was almost always followed by a walk on the dock. One of Charlotte's hands clutched her father's and the other an ice cream cone—their mutual favorite, mint chocolate chip. They'd stroll through the park, beneath a canopy of trees, and watch teenagers play a pick-up game on the basketball courts or wave to sailboats from the deck of the pavilion at sunset. Elise had usually walked a bit behind, allowing them their rare father-daughter moments.

Charlotte wove her way back to Second Street and exited the east gate. She spotted the ferry in the distance, churning its way north toward Kelleys Island. Driving through a residential area, she popped out onto the main road leading into Marblehead, and her foot automatically lifted off the gas as she crossed beneath the quarry overpass. There was always a decent chance a police cruiser would lie in wait just beyond.

She passed the senior living center where Anne Sutton—Chuck's mother from whom Charlotte received her middle name—lived out her final days as a dementia patient in the memory care unit. She'd not returned for Grandmother Sutton's funeral the summer after moving to Pittsburgh. It had been too soon after her abrupt departure, and they'd never been close, despite living in the same community.

Anne Sutton had been just as into sports as Chuck and would have loved having a grandson. Charlotte groaned. Her grandmother hadn't crossed her mind in years, until now, and really, how much more guilt could she pile on her own plate? She'd been in the dark about Adam as much as anyone. It wasn't her fault. She'd had nothing to do with any of it.

Just after the municipal building, she slowed to catch a glimpse of The Clip Joint, formerly the House of Beauty and her go-to salon. A glimmer of light shone through the windows, but the sign in the window read "CLOSED." She glanced down at her phone. 11:43 a.m. If Sammy did business on a Sunday, he'd probably start at noon.

Passing several shops, restaurants, and a winery housed in an old, stone schoolhouse, Charlotte took a left at the sign for the

Marblehead Lighthouse, and wound down a lane to the point. She drove around the circle and pulled parallel to the water, idling for a moment before cutting the ignition.

The lighthouse, a white monolith of sandstone originally constructed back in the early 1800s, had been one of her and Sammy's favorite spots to sit and gossip about their classmates or, in Charlotte's case mostly, scheme about getting out of small-town Ohio. They'd even had their first kiss there, ending in giggles instead of fireworks. They'd flirted with a relationship in high school, holding hands as boyfriend and girlfriend for an afternoon, but the experiment led to laughter in the halls and more than a few jokes about Sammy's sexuality and Charlotte's height. Too much drama for both of them. After several awkward apologies, and a full week of each avoiding the other, they'd returned to being best friends.

Nothing more.

Charlotte wouldn't have made it through high school without Sammy. Whatever the state of their friendship, Sammy was *her* Sammy, and she'd missed him. He'd never given her any reason to leave, and he'd always been there for her. Certainly, more than her father.

Chuck had rarely given her a reason to stay.

A lump formed in Charlotte's stomach. She couldn't—wouldn't—be Power of Attorney for him. And certainly not guardian to Adam. It was too much. She resented the ask.

Creeping from the vehicle, she wandered down the path toward the water and picked up a rock, cold and hard in her palm. She cocked her arm back and let it go with a grunt. A ghost of knowledge passed down from her father. Instead of skipping across the water, it landed with a plop about six feet from shore.

Unsatisfying.

Brushing her palm on her jeans, Charlotte returned to her car. It was half past noon.

Why not? She'd stop and surprise Sammy. He'd listen; he'd always been available when she needed him, and she was 100% sure she needed him now.

Charlotte pulled out and, within minutes, parked in front of The Clip Joint. It looked entirely different than it had when she was a child. Sammy from Miami had painted the brick surrounding the salon door a vibrant turquoise with an orange stripe—Miami Dolphins colors. Never mind that he had lived in Browns country for more than 15 years. Sammy's inspiration bloomed from whatever source he wished. Public opinion never swayed him; she loved that about him.

Through the large, street-front windows, Charlotte spotted her best friend, the 10-years-older Sammy, dressed in his usual black and snipping away at the blue-gray bob of some matronly type. She put her hand to her mouth as he shimmied from side to side, a blur of motion. Charlotte couldn't see his feet, but assumed his only hint of color was a pair of bright red sneakers. He'd be providing his customer with a steady stream of flirtatious compliments and fishing tips or, just as likely, humming to a favorite 80s song playing in the background. Certain things weren't meant to change; Sammy was one of them. Charlotte sighed, a weight lifting from her heart. Perhaps, at least *one* good thing would come of her trip.

Oh, dude. I've missed you.

From the back, Sammy's client—a woman dressed in a fuchsia, velour jogging suit—appeared to have fallen asleep in the chair.

Charlotte paused to take in the welcome mat, featuring a picture of a Sammy-lookalike holding a cigarette with one hand and combing his black hair in a mirror with the other. A hazy graphic of smoke and psychedelic colors swirled around the words "The Clip Joint."

Socially unapologetic and hilariously Sammy.

A faint tinkle of bells preceded her as Charlotte opened the door. Sammy turned with a shake of his hips, and his dance moves came to a grinding halt.

"Hello, Sammy," Charlotte whispered.

There was no expression on Sammy's face. None.

Charlotte felt rooted to the spot. Unable to move forward. Unable to step back out the door as if she'd never come.

Sammy turned his back to the door. "Mama? Mama, come to the front. We've got a visitor." He looked down at the blue-gray bob and resumed his cutting. "Almost done, Mrs. T. Lookin' like the catch of the day, like always."

With more force than necessary, he shoved a cord into the socket by his mirror and started the blow dryer. The whine of the motor sounded like a small twin-engine taking off from the Erie-Ottawa International Airport.

"Sammy?" Charlotte raised her voice.

Sammy adjusted the setting of the blow dryer to "high."

"Sammy!"

"Mama, come to the front," Sammy said.

Mrs. Macon scurried from the back room. As short and thin as her son, the smiling Latino woman held a broom in one hand and a plate of cookies in the other.

"Would our visitor like a cookie?" she said with a barely perceptible accent. Mrs. Macon held the tray toward Charlotte.

"Hi, Mama Macon."

"Charlotte? Wait, what? Sammy, it's Charlotte." Plunking the tray on the nearby reception desk, Mrs. Macon threw her tiny arms around Charlotte's waist.

Here we go.

"Our beautiful girl."

Mrs. Macon's arms grew tighter. Warmth radiating through her, Charlotte patted the woman gingerly on the back and pulled back to put at least an inch or two between them. "Oh, Mama, it's so good to see you, too." She shifted closer to the cookie tray. "Are those polvorones? Your shortbread? Oh, my god. I love your shortbread. *Always* my favorite."

"But you didn't call my Sammy." Mrs. Macon suddenly swept the tray of cookies out from under Charlotte's wavering hand. "You didn't call." A stream of Spanish, all of which Charlotte was very glad she didn't understand, filled the air with sharp syllables and anxious vowels. Mrs. Macon only ever reverted to her native tongue when she was upset. It was a fact.

"I'm sorry—"

"Why didn't you call Sammy? You ran off to the big city and left my boy. What's wrong with you, child? Sammy is a catch. How am I ever going to become a grandmother when you do a thing like that? Hmmm?" Mrs. Macon's pleasure at seeing Charlotte had turned to an inquisition in less time than it took to say polvorones.

"Es estupido," Mama Macon muttered, beneath the whine of the blow dryer.

Sammy turned off the device and spun his client around to face the door, revealing a woman with piercing eyes trained on Charlotte. Rhinestone-speckled readers hung from a chain around her neck, and an obese Chihuahua dressed in a purple vest and rhinestone collar sat on the woman's lap. Its eyes bulged, watching Charlotte's every move. Sammy aimed an equally unhappy glare in her direction.

"I'm so sorry. Please, Sammy," Charlotte pleaded. "I didn't stay in touch with anyone. When I left, I just wanted to forget this place."

Bobbed Mrs. T listened with the attention span of the town's biggest gossip. Her bejeweled fingers stroked the Chihuahua, making its eyes bug out even more.

"I didn't mean to upset anyone. I just wanted to leave." Charlotte's voice dipped to a whisper. "I'm sorry. I never thought I'd come back."

Sammy's gaze was trained on the top of Mrs. T's head.

"Phhtt," Mrs. Macon said. "Friends need friends." Mama Macon swung the cookie tray back around and jabbed Charlotte in the stomach with it. "Well, at least you're here now, child. Small grace that it is. Eat. Eat."

Charlotte grabbed a shortbread. It melted in her mouth as Sammy removed the cape from around his client's neck. Using a towel, he brushed away some stray hairs—DNA orphans sent to their doom on black and white checked tiles.

"Did you need me to take a straightener to this, Mrs. T?" Sammy said. "A little hairspray before you break every heart in Marble-head?"

"My heartbreaking days are long past, dear." Mrs. T. smiled as she dug her fingers into the bob and pulled the strands toward her cheeks. Puckering her lips, she turned this way and that. "No, Sammy, honey. No hairspray. This'll do just fine. Won't it, Snuggles?" Lifting the dog, she waved its paw at her reflection in the mirror. "Yes, it will. It'll do juuust fine." Mrs. T slipped a wad of tip money into Sammy's palm and patted the back of his tattooed hand. "Now don't forget to come to the Thanksgiving potluck, dear. I'm making my apple dumplings just for you."

"Wouldn't miss it for anything," Sammy said.

"I should introduce you to my niece." Mrs. T nodded at Mama Macon. "Cute little blonde. She just moved back to town. Good birthing hips like the rest of the women in my family, if it's grand-children you're wanting."

"Sweet of you," Mrs. Macon said.

Sammy's eyes widened. "Wow, Mrs. T. I don't know what to say."

Mrs. T shook her bedazzled purse, releasing some stray hairs, and waltzed to the reception desk.

"Excuse me." She threw the purse onto the counter with a thump and, standing too close, gave Charlotte a thorough onceover. Charlotte backed away, and Mrs. Macon's fingernails sailed over the keys of a calculator.

Mrs. T gave Charlotte another look, longer this time.

"I'm an old friend." Charlotte shrugged and turned. "Sammy, can we please talk? I need—"

But Sammy was gone.

Presumably in the back, with his anger and his pride.

"Sammy?"

There was no answer. Charlotte turned toward Mama Macon.

"Seriously? This is ridiculous."

90

"Dear goodness." Mrs. T shook her head. "Have a nice day, Maria." She tucked her pooch under one arm, purse under the other, and departed, letting the door slam back on its hinge with a flourish and tinkle.

"Sammy, don't be rude. Come," Mama Macon said, her wrath displayed in just five little words.

Charlotte frowned. "I don't—"

"You'll have to excuse my baby, Charlotte. You broke his heart. Come, Sammy."

Sammy did not come. It was probably the first time in 28 years he'd disobeyed a direct order from his mother, and he'd be in serious trouble for it later. No one defied Mama Macon without a sizeable amount of risk.

Shit. He's really pissed.

"Try again tomorrow, sweet girl."

Charlotte nodded.

"Thanks, Mama."

"It'll be all right. It's not too late. You're both still plenty young enough to give me grandbabies. What would Sammy want with a cute little blonde, anyway? He has you."

"I'm sure Sammy will give you a grandbaby someday, but not likely with me." Charlotte hesitated, looking toward the door leading to the back room. "I'm sorry... for everything."

"It'll be all right. I promise."

"I doubt it."

Charlotte sighed. Her best friend—the one person she'd always counted on and experienced so many firsts with—had been holding on to a 10-year-old hurt just like she had. She was the reason. Instead of finding comfort in her visit, it had ended almost as badly as her weekend began.

What have I done?

Charlotte exited the salon and hopped over The Clip Joint welcome mat in an act of defiance.

Or deference. She wasn't sure which.

11

HIGH SCHOOL

Fifteen-year-old Charlotte dropped down on her bed.

"If I'm going to do this, it has to be you, Sammy."

"You sure?" Sammy lay beside her, his hands clasped behind his head as he stared up at the bedroom ceiling. He wore a Billy Joel concert tee, from which he'd cut the arms. A tattoo of sheet music rippled up his bicep. Red sneakers and scrawny ankles poked out from the cuff of his jeans.

"I'm sure," Charlotte said.

"We get caught, Elise is going to lose her shit."

"I don't care." Charlotte nudged his ribs with her elbow. "It's my body, and I can do what I want with it. Besides, Mom won't be home for another hour."

"'Kay, if you say so. Sammy from Miami, at your service." The boy rolled off the bed and gathered the supplies he always kept in his backpack, just in case.

"Towel?"

Charlotte motioned to a beach towel hanging on her bedpost.

"Trashcan?"

Charlotte nodded toward her desk.

"Let's do this thing," Sammy said. "Maybe in front of the mirror? So you can watch?"

"I guess, but I'm a little... "

"Scared? Yeah. Me too." Sammy shrugged. "It's all good, man."

Charlotte crawled from the bed and approached the full-length mirror hanging on the back of her bedroom door. She sat on the edge of her chair. With a flourish, Sammy threw the towel around Charlotte's shoulders and placed the trashcan in her lap.

"Hold, Char."

"You're so demanding." Charlotte *didn't* want to watch. She *was* scared. Maybe more than she wanted to admit.

"Do it," she said, closing her eyes.

Seconds ticked by. Nothing happened. She opened her left lid, keeping the right firmly shut, and met Sammy's stoic gaze in the mirror.

"Dude, seriously. Get on with it, or I'll chicken out. What are you waiting for?"

"A miracle?" Sammy grasped a long chunk of Charlotte's wavy hair and fanned the strands under his nose, forming a black, bushy mass. "What mustache I do with this mess?"

"I don't know," Charlotte said. "Whatever you think."

"You've got to give me more than *that*. You sure you don't want Mary Lou at the House of Beauty to cut it, Char? I'm feeling pressure. Sammy doesn't like pressure."

Charlotte rolled her eyes. "Come on. I want my best friend to do it, as long as he stops talking about himself in the third person. You're overthinking it. It's not calculus."

"Pressure," Sammy grunted.

"Don't be such a wimp. I have an idea." Charlotte swept her hair away from her face and pulled it into a high ponytail using a rubber band from a collection around her wrist. Loosening the pony, she deftly braided the hair and fastened it at the bottom with another band. She dropped her hands into her lap. "Easy. Just chop the damn thing off."

In the mirror, Sammy's startled brown eyes met Charlotte's now calm ones.

"All of it?"

"Yes, all of it."

"Um, there's, like, at least a foot—"

"All of it, Sammy. I've made up my mind."

"If you say so." Cocking his head, Sammy raised a pair of scissors and snipped the braid off at the base, just above the band. He held it up to the light and dropped the offering into Charlotte's waiting palm. "There. You can donate it."

"Oh." Charlotte's jaw dropped. The coarse strands of the braid tickled her fingers. It was so long. She stared at Sammy in the mirror; his eyes were as large as golf balls.

"Char? You made me do it," Sammy whispered. "You told me to."

"Yeah." Charlotte gazed at her reflection. The heavy braid fell into the trash, and she tentatively reached up and ran her fingers through the short tufts framing her heart-shaped face. She wasn't sure what to think.

"Well?" Sammy tilted his head to one side. "Maybe let me clean it up a bit?"

"Yeah."

With a snip here and a snip there, Sammy added layering and trimmed it even tighter at the base of Charlotte's neck and above her ears. The snip of the scissors grew in volume and speed. Finally, he stepped back from his work and swept the towel from Charlotte's shoulders.

"Nailed it." There was a gleam in Sammy's eyes.

"Holy crap, Sammy."

"Is that a good holy crap or a bad holy crap?"

"I... don't know." Flipping over at the waist, Charlotte ruffled the feathery cap, dislodging more hairs and sending them winging through the room. She raised her head and looked again into the mirror. Her eyes, with noticeable flecks of gold around the irises, seemed brighter. Bigger. The freckles across her nose were still prominent, more so than before. Charlotte didn't even mind her neck, long and smooth, fully exposed now, rising out of her hoodie like a lone flower stem poking up through the mulch.

Somehow, the pixie cut worked.

Charlotte smiled. "It will take some getting used to, but I love it. Thank you."

"You look dope as hell." Sammy shook his head. "Like a model."

"Not hardly."

"Hardly," Sammy said, an odd tenor to his voice. "Verrry hardly."

"What's that supposed to mean?"

"Nothing." Sammy shook the towel over the trash can and folded it. When his glance met hers, his cheeks were red.

"Are you—?"

"Should I be?"

"No," Charlotte said. "At least I don't think so."

"Yeah. Okay, then," Sammy said. "Elise is going to birth a cow, isn't she?"

"Yep. Maybe we don't tell her you did it."

12

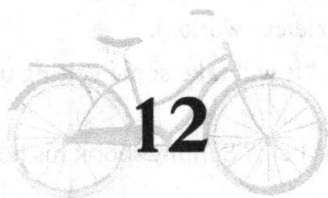

Charlotte pulled onto Main Street. How much more could she take? It was worse than dealing with her father. At least with Chuck, Charlotte expected disappointment. With Sammy, she'd always had someone to lean on.

Until now.

When she and her mother left Lakeside, she'd never considered how Sammy might feel. She'd assumed he'd move on to bigger and better things, just as she had. No matter how much Mama Macon had wanted it, it's not like they'd loved each other. Well, not that way. She'd loved Sammy, but she hadn't been *in* love with him. They'd only ever been the best of friends. They'd done everything together. Always together.

How can he be so mad? Sammy's never mad.

Not ready to return to Sutton's Choice, Charlotte drove out of town. It wasn't long before she realized her path was leading her past every one of her and Sammy's favorite haunts.

Netty's, where they'd eaten chili dogs.

Check.

East Harbor State Park, where they'd swam off the beach; African Safari Wildlife Park, where they'd ridden camels; Cheese Haven, where they'd sampled every cheese.

Check. Check. Check.

Letting the memories take over—and feeling more and more sorry for herself—she approached a gas station and flicked her fingers in a half-hearted wave to "Handless Jacques," a 28-foot-tall fiberglass promotional figure in the side yard.

Then did a double-take.

Barely slowing down, she swerved into the empty parking lot and came to an abrupt halt beside the statue that had originally served as a sandwich shop mascot. Affectionately called the Maitre d' of Marblehead, the mustachioed fellow wore a tailcoat, red bow tie, and a chef's hat, his dark, jacketed arms thrust out in supplication.

"Whoa. You've finally got hands."

Charlotte remembered Jacques in a terrible state of disrepair with faded paint, broken coat tails, a sizeable hole in his pants in a very unfortunate location, and holding nothing more than empty bars of rusted pylon—a sad figure missing not just its digits but a tray of treats. As a child, Charlotte had nightmares of Jacques coming to life and strolling, willy-nilly, through the streets of Lakeside—always ending with his giant foot stepping on their cottage and squashing her inside the old structure.

Charlotte smiled. "Not so scary now, are you, buddy?" He'd been handless her entire youth, but while she was gone, someone had renovated the statue with a fresh coat of paint and a large set of white-gloved appendages—new again, friendly and welcoming, like he was just waiting for a handshake.

She bet Sammy absolutely *loved* the upgrade.

During their senior year, they had given the big guy an overnight makeover for the holidays. Wrapped in red from head to toe and sporting a fake beard, Jacques made a magnificent Santa. Sammy had even climbed onto Charlotte's shoulders and added a colorful Christmas package to hold. Rumors had circulated that the football

97

team had done it as a harmless holiday prank, but the theory had never been proven and no one had officially claimed it. Charlotte grinned. She and Sammy had been more than happy to let the athletes take the credit, since to confess to the deed would have meant certain punishment.

Charlotte peered up at Jacques. Her eyes burned with unshed tears.

Senior stunt.

Check.

How can Sammy be so mad?

Swiping at her cheek, Charlotte said a silent "goodbye" to no-longer-handless Jacques and a silent "sorry" to her best friend.

* * * * *

That afternoon, Franco Bellimer waved her over to his Sunday football table of choice, the one in the corner closest to the big-screen TV. In front of Charlotte's high school mentor sat a mounded platter of nachos supreme and a pitcher of piss-yellow lite beer, taking up most of the tabletop. Three empty shot glasses squatted in an orderly row beside his silverware.

"Glad you could join me," Franco said, vaguely motioning to the stool beside him. "Sit. Sit. But first, I need to give you a hug and proper condolences." He reached out and awkwardly placed an arm around Charlotte's shoulder, pulling her in.

Charlotte didn't want to overanalyze the warmth of his gesture. She'd missed him, too. Almost as much as Sammy. It had been so easy to walk away from Lakeside and its many characters. The return was not nearly so painless.

"I'm sorry. This must all be so hard for you," Bellimer said.

His voice was gruff from years of chain-smoking. He carried with him the distinctive odor of unfiltered cigarettes, sucked to the husk and discarded as white, charred little nubs. The smell had never bothered Charlotte. She'd always found Bellimer's faint smoky odor, mixed with a hint of sweat, somewhat comforting.

Charlotte inched down onto a stool. "Thanks, Mr. B."

"Thank *you* for taking the time for a chat." Bellimer played with a chip and twirled some cheese. "We certainly need one."

"Sure."

Charlotte didn't know what to expect, but she had a vague feeling she wasn't going to like it. Similar to the stop at The Clip Joint, this meeting with an old friend would likely not go her way. She could feel it. Mr. B sounded primed for a lecture.

He tapped a nacho on the side of the plate, dislodging an excess of black olives, and glanced in the direction of Bea filling a beer at the tap.

"You'd think by now that nutty, old cougar would know I hate olives," he said. "Sometimes I think she aims to vex me."

Charlotte's mouth twitched.

"Anyway, since you're leaving again so quickly, I guess I better cut to the chase. We both know Chuck is a very smart man."

"He is."

"Just my opinion, but I'm pretty sure his health is 100 times worse than he lets on."

"What do you mean?"

"He's been compensating for his memory losses, like with the sticky notes, for a long time. I think the Alzheimer's, if that's what this is... and I suspect it is... has progressed much further than we realize." Bellimer shrugged. "Maybe the rest of us just didn't see the signs early enough. My aunt went through this. Trust me. It happens."

"I really don't know anything about Alzheimer's," Charlotte mumbled.

"Then research it. You're good at that," Bellimer said. "He can't drive anymore, or, I should say, he shouldn't. Still does, though. Discuss it with his doctor. She'll help. Chuck is as stubborn as you are, so it may take some convincing to get him to give up his keys. He'll have more medical appointments to schedule, and he shouldn't be driving himself. You'll need to talk some sense into your father about, well, a lot of things. Go back to Pittsburgh and get your affairs in order, but return as soon as possible, Charlotte. There's a lot to deal with."

Charlotte chose her words carefully. "Like I said yesterday, I'm just taking Chuck to his neurology appointment. I can't come back soon. I've got a job with an advertising agency."

Franco Bellimer's brows arched. His eyes grew small, and the silence between them stretched.

"I'm sorry, Mr. B. I just can't. I don't want to lose my job."

"I see. Well, that is certainly understandable." Bellimer hesitated. "But you'll be coming back regularly, though, right? To take your father to his appointments?"

"Not that I'd planned. I'm just here to get things in order."

"It's not that simple nor that quick. There's a lot to deal with. Your father isn't the only thing that's failing here. So's the paper." Franco Bellimer took a sip of beer. "He's missed some steps. It's a real shame. There aren't too many community papers still in business, but everyone relies on *The Lakeside Line.* I'm doing all I can for him, but your dad is a proud man. He's having a hard time with all this. I assumed you'd help him and Adam get through it."

Charlotte sucked in a breath. "Considering I just found out I *have* a brother, I don't see how you could have assumed any such thing. No offense, Mr. B, but I didn't want to come back, and now I have even less interest in staying."

Franco Bellimer's small eyes grew smaller.

"I just came because I was expected to. I know that sounds bad, but it's true." It bothered Charlotte that she had to justify her feelings to one of the few people she'd thought would understand. "It's not like my dad even stayed in touch with me."

"Yes, I suppose there's that."

"Besides, people around here never much liked me, and I never much liked them. I don't want to be here. I didn't ask for any of this."

"You think Chuck did? No one asks for this. He's ill. And he's not getting better. You're a reasonable person... or you used to be. I hoped you'd gotten over old, petty nonsense from your youth, by now. Maybe see past what's ailing you to what is ailing the rest of your family."

The rebuke felt like a slap to the face. Charlotte was right back in high school, sent to the principal's office because of something someone else had done. Somehow, Charlotte had become the problem, not Sammy or Dana or Franco Bellimer. And certainly not Chuck. Never Chuck.

"My family is complicated."

"You think I don't know that? Join the club. Everybody's family is complicated. Don't be shy, child." Bellimer softened the blow by pushing the nachos toward her. "I need these like a heart attack."

Charlotte glanced down at the bribe.

"Look, I like you, Charlotte. I always have," Bellimer said. "I loved the writing you did in my class. Now that you're all grown up, I read your essays every time you're published. I am so proud of all you've accomplished. I get that you don't want to lose your job, and you don't want to be back here. You struggled with a lot of teen demons. That's what this is really about. Teenagers can be cruel. I even witnessed a few things in my classroom. I get it. I really do. Hell, I've been in your shoes. You think someone who looks like me had an easy time of it when I was a kid? They called me Jelly Belly. Belly for short."

"I don't—"

"Let me finish." Bellimer jabbed a nacho in the air. "This isn't just about a few high school bullies. I know your family life wasn't exactly rainbows and kittens. Your dad could have done better. A lot better, if I'm frank. Growing up must have been a real struggle."

"Exactly."

Bellimer took his time shoving a chip between his teeth. Charlotte's stomach clenched. She waited for the "but."

"I get all of it, *but* Chuck's the one who is struggling now, and you need to be the bigger person. Stop feeling sorry for yourself and make peace with your pop. Family is still family, and family comes first. Reconsider and stick around, for a while. To be frank, you may not have much longer to reconcile things with Chuck. Or this community, for that matter. Just my opinion, for what it's worth."

A chip turned to sawdust in Charlotte's mouth. "Your opinion has always meant a lot to me, Mr. B."

"Good. Then listen up. I put it at a year, probably less, and Chuck's going to be unable to run the business. You're a very good writer. It would be a shame to see your legacy just left on the cutting room floor."

Charlotte pulled another nacho from the mix, the cheese stringing its way from platter to chip, a slippery rope. She scanned the television screens, all featuring Cleveland losing to Denver, 21-0. At the end of the bar, a man frowned at the beer in front of him. She supposed it was that kind of day.

"Why do you call it my legacy? It's not." Charlotte's voice was barely audible, even to her own ears. "A legacy is something one family member hands down to another. My father never cared about my writing. He wanted me to be an athlete, not a writer." Charlotte's voice rose. In that moment, she finally understood her father, and she despised him for it. "He wanted to be the only writer in our family."

Bellimer sighed. "Do you hear yourself?"

Charlotte eyed her mentor. She sounded childish—jealous, even—but it was a relief to put into words the hurt she'd felt not being included in Chuck's successes or in his life. Charlotte was invisible to him. He'd preferred touring and screwing fans like Sophia, instead of being with his own family.

"I hear," Charlotte said clearly. "And I don't give a damn how I sound. I don't give a damn about Chuck's paper either."

"Harsh words, considering he wants you to run it someday—to take over."

Charlotte slumped back in her chair. "That's ridiculous. The paper is just an expensive hobby to him."

"I don't think so. He's built his business up to be handed down to his children. He just didn't expect to have to do it this soon."

"You're wrong." Charlotte snapped up another nacho, shoving the whole thing in her mouth. "My father told me he didn't even want children."

"I see."

"Holy H. Hell," Bea shouted. Charlotte's gaze slid to the television. Cleveland had fumbled at the goal line. A series of groans circulated around the room, and a Denver fan, isolated in his oneness, threw up his hands in excitement, only to be shushed by his partner dressed in orange and brown.

"Charlotte, what is it that you want?" Bellimer said. "When it comes to your dad, what do you hope for? Why *did* you come to Ohio if you didn't expect to get something out of it? Or at least stay to help? Why did you come? Can you even answer the question?"

"I don't understand what you mean." Charlotte frowned. "I felt obligated to come. I wasn't expecting anything at all."

"You sure about that?" Bellimer scratched his bald head then rubbed it, searching for phantom hairs still residing there. "You didn't come all this way—"

"I'm here because it's expected of me," Charlotte said. "That's it. That's all. My dad is sick. I did what any good daughter would do. I came home because I didn't have a choice."

"You always have a choice," Bellimer said. "You could have chosen *not* to come, but you did. You get to decide what you walk away from this with—comfort, regret, answers? Whatever. You *do* have a choice. But you need to recognize it is your father who doesn't. Sure, he made some questionable choices when you were young. Ones I would hope I would never have made myself, under the same circumstances. It doesn't mean that he doesn't regret those choices. We all have made choices we regret. I just don't want you to regret the ones you make now. Bad choices can haunt you for the rest of your life."

Charlotte's emotions had formed into a hard, little lump. Unsettled. Off balance.

"Choices are like relatives, Charlotte. We all have them, but some are more appealing than others." Bellimer shrugged. "Sometimes, it's the unsavory ones we have to cozy up to, for the good of the situation. Not much different than embracing my cousin Eddy. He's the slacker in the family, and not too bright, but he has a mighty fine fishing boat, beer in the fridge, and a great sense of humor, which usually includes fart jokes. I still see the value in choosing Eddy on a sunny afternoon."

The entire bar went bananas.

"Well, there's a pleasant change." Franco spun the platter of chips. "We just intercepted a pass."

Nothing really changes.

Not really.

13

HIGH SCHOOL

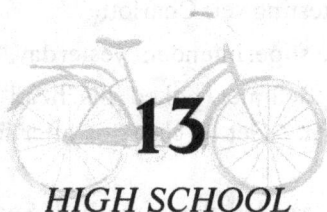

"9-1-1, what is your hair emergency?"

Charlotte rifled through her sophomore locker, fumbling for her journalism journal and advanced English book.

"The Tree got trimmed."

"They have extensions for that."

The familiar voices, pure snark, trailed off. Pulling on the short waves tickling her neck, Charlotte turned in time to see Dana and Nicki descend the stairs in a fit of giggles, their backsides swishing inside the skin-tight sausage casings they called cheer skirts. How anyone was supposed to do a split in those things was beyond Charlotte's comprehension. Nicki's skirt was wider. Birthing hips, Charlotte's mother would have said.

"Feel sorry for them, Char," Sammy said, nudging her on his way past. "They're sharing one brain."

"If that," Charlotte said. "Hurry. We don't want to be late, or Mr. B will make us do the final line edits on the Thursday edition."

Charlotte and Sammy slipped into the classroom just as Franco Bellimer took his usual spot on the corner of his desk. The man's stubby little legs swung stubby little feet back and forth. He dabbed his bald head and defogged his glasses with a handkerchief he kept tucked up one jacket sleeve.

"Nice of you to join us, Miss Sutton. Mr. Macon."

"Sorry, Mr. B," Charlotte and Sammy said in unison.

"By the skin of your teeth. I'll let it slide, just this once." Mr. Bellimer jumped down from his perch and grabbed the attendance checklist on a clipboard by the door. "Did you get to that article about standardized testing yet, Charlotte?"

"I interviewed the superintendent yesterday."

"Excellent." Mr. Bellimer poked his head out the door and looked left, then right. "Get to class, or after-school detention for all of you."

Muffled laughter traveled down the hall. Some kids showed up to Bellimer's detention, even if they'd done nothing wrong. The newspaper staff did a lot of its work after school, in the back of his classroom, while the front of the room served as the holding cell for the "educationally detained." Detention usually entailed folding newspapers or selling copies at whatever sporting or special event was going on in the school after hours. As long as everyone was doing something productive, Bellimer made it an after-school social hour.

"Pull up a chair, and let's see what else we've got. Sammy?"

"'Kay, the feature about the spring dance is almost finished, and the advice column only had three questions this week."

Kate Fallow added, "I took photos of our Teacher of the Week, did an article on gender-neutral bathrooms, and finished my opinion piece about the crappy cafeteria food."

"Excellent," Bellimer said. "I'm sure it will be, er, appetizing. What about you, Jenny?"

Jenny Kim covered the basics of two sports articles—the promising start for the boys' basketball team and the lack of funding to add a girls' field hockey team.

Dana and Nicki whispered from their desks in the back.

"Something you'd like to share, ladies?" the teacher said, raising a brow.

Nicki's nasal voice slid to a high-pitched whine. "What's the point of field hockey, Mr. B? I mean, there were only, like, a dozen girls interested or something. Like, what's the big deal? It's a butch sport, anyway. Gross."

"I was one of those dozen girls." Jenny stood and crossed her arms. "Are you calling me 'butch'? So, what if I am?"

"You're not butch." Grant Warren's pimply face turned a red-der-than-average shade. "And definitely not gross. Not gross at all."

An awkward moment of silence followed. Mr. Bellimer cleared his throat.

"Out of line, Nicki. Perhaps you'd like to work on the final edits for the Thursday paper?"

"Like, no thanks."

"Let me rephrase that, not in the form of a question. You and Dana *will* do the final line edits, while everyone else takes stock of the advertisements that came in this week." Mr. Bellimer motioned to the class with a dismissive wave. "Go ahead and get started. Charlotte, may I speak with you in my office for a moment?"

"What did you do?" Sammy whispered.

Charlotte frowned. "Nothing I know of."

"We'll only be a minute," Bellimer said. "Work on your own."

Charlotte followed Mr. Bellimer into his clear-glassed cubicle. She took a seat with her back to the window facing the classroom. Every single student would be staring a hole through the glass. She could almost feel it.

"Nosy buggers." Bellimer crossed behind Charlotte. "Get to work, you lot, or it's after-school detention for all of you."

Charlotte's lips twitched as a chorus of "Yes, Mr. B" filtered back. He closed the door.

"Sorry," Mr. Bellimer said. "I didn't mean to give them grist for the mill."

"It's okay. What's up, Mr. B?"

"I have a favor to ask. Do you think your father would mind talking to the journalism and English classes? I'm in charge of getting speakers for Career Day in April."

"Oh." Charlotte nodded, relieved she'd done nothing wrong. "Sure. I'll ask him, but he travels a lot."

"His story could be really inspiring for the kids. To have access to a published author or professional athlete is unusual, any day, but that we have both in the same person? I'd love to include him, if he's not too busy."

He's always too busy.

"Sure. No problem. I'll ask."

"Thank you. And have you had the chance to think any more about the personal essay column I hope to add next month? It would be a great fit for you."

"Yeah, I guess," Charlotte said, "but I don't have any idea what to write about. It's called 'personal' for reasons, you know?"

"I respect that."

"Anyway, I doubt anyone wants to hear my stories. They aren't as interesting as my dad's, if that's what you're thinking."

"No one expects you to write like your father," Mr. Bellimer said. He frowned, shaking his head. "You are you, and Chuck is Chuck. What you have to say, and how you do so, is different from your dad, but just as interesting. I want to hear *your* stories. You're one of my brightest journalism students, Charlotte. Maybe the best young writer who has come through my door. This would be a great opportunity for you."

Charlotte sat straighter in her chair. Mr. B liked her writing.

"A chip off your father's block, I'd say. You could make writing a career, too, if you wanted. Anyway, I'd really like to feature your work in the essay column. Please, give it some thought."

He'd actually noticed. Charlotte smiled.

"Okay."

"Excellent. And don't forget to let me know if we can add your father to the Career Day speaker list."

"I'll ask him, but he's really busy."

14

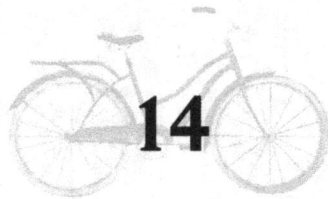

Forming an uncomfortable and unspoken truce, Chuck and Charlotte decided to return, together, to the newspaper office early on Monday morning.

"I took your suggestion and went to see Sammy yesterday," Charlotte said, walking beside Chuck along the waterfront path. "It went horribly."

"I'm sorry to hear that, Charlie."

"You were right. He was really mad. I've never seen him like that. Ever."

Chuck simply patted his daughter on the shoulder. Charlotte took it as a sign of sympathy, something he had not been particularly good at showing when she was a child. It had always been about being tough, picking yourself up, and trying again, something she could remember doing a lot of on and off the field.

As Chuck swung open the gate and motioned her through, Charlotte noticed the *Erie Mermaid* floating at the end of the dock.

"I wonder if Jake has any charters today."

"I don't know. Would you like him to stop in so you can ask him?"

"Hmmph. I'd just like a chance to pet Sydney."

"What?"

"His dog?"

"Oh, right. Sydney. Great dog."

Charlotte followed her father into the office, and Chuck immediately sat down and scanned his notes.

"I think we should go through as much as possible, so someone other than just Franco knows what's going on around here," he said. "You're my daughter, and you'll need to know what's what when my memory completely goes. Or worse. I strike out once and for all."

Charlotte rolled her shoulders, feeling the tension build.

Don't let him get to you.

Charlotte's father sighed. "I'm probably down to my last out, kid. Bottom of the ninth. It's time to step up—"

"Lose the sports bullshit, Chuck. If you're going to play the death card—"

"Sorry," Chuck said softly.

The usual guilt crept to the surface. She had no patience, nor could she fathom where to find some.

"It's fine. Let's see what you've got." Charlotte leaned over the work table. Different-colored notes lined the surface in six rows of eight—neat and orderly—precisely where her father had made them come to attention like little paper soldiers on a battlefield. A single pink note, in the upper right corner, said "CHARLIE (daughter), legal papers, bottom file drawer."

Notes on yellow indicated appointments and general to-dos, and notes on green represented due-dates for bills, printing deadlines, etc. A separate sheet of paper, taped in the left corner, included names and contact info squeezed into every margin. Charlotte's own name graced the top, along with her current phone number and correct apartment address. Charlotte assumed her mother must have given it to him after college graduation. She certainly had not. With her diploma, she had considered herself independent from her father—financially, emotionally, physically. Off the Chuck grid.

"Huh. You've really got a system." Charlotte surreptitiously took a picture of the contact list with her phone.

Chuck shrugged, perusing his many notes. "I've used the same system for years—ever since I took over this place, really. It's become all the more important, recently."

They spent the next two hours going through files, checking Chuck's deadlines, and reconciling the stories and advertising going into the next issue. Charlotte found herself listening closely. It was, as far back as she could remember, the first time they had ever spent such a long time together doing something of which they could both relate. For some reason, the thought filled Charlotte with an acute sadness she couldn't explain and didn't want to analyze.

"Who lays out the copy for you?" she said.

Chuck pointed to the vacant office. "I hired Kate Fallow, a few years back. She does a lot remotely. She's also my photographer when I need one."

"Really?" Charlotte smiled. "Kate was in my journalism class. A year behind me, maybe two?"

Chuck nodded. "She's really good. I only use her two days a week for the layout and final copyediting. Our advertising has slipped recently. Everything is so digital now. People don't want to pay for advertising in a newspaper when they can use social media for free online, I suppose."

Or her father's illness had something to do with losing advertisers.

Chuck pulled a paper from his in-box, scanned it, and transferred the information onto an appropriately colored note. Crumpling the original paper into a ball, he overhanded it into the basketball hoop across the room. It fell into the trashcan beneath without touching the rim.

"Two points."

Charlotte shook her head. "I can't believe you still have that old hoop."

"Old man. Old hoop. Old habits."

"You're not that old, Chuck. What are you? 53? 54?"

"I'm 55, but I feel older. Ancient, sometimes, when I can't remember something."

"I bet." From what Charlotte had read about Alzheimer's, it was more common in people over 65. Her father would fall into the category of "early-onset"—particularly cruel that he would lose his mental abilities when his body was still so young and able.

Bending over her father's computer, Charlotte shook the mouse to wake the screen. "About your advertising... maybe what you need is to step up your own digital presence. Social media doesn't have to be a bad thing. What's your web address?"

Chuck raised his eyebrows. "You don't know?"

"No. Should I?" She'd never been on her father's website, not even for voyeuristic purposes. He'd taken the paper after she left, and she just hadn't cared enough to snoop. His successes had been in her face all during her growing-up years, and she had her own writing to think about now. His didn't matter. Not to her. Not like it should.

Chuck grabbed a note from his desk, keeping a finger in its place. "I don't know it either." He thrust a paper with the web address under Charlotte's nose. Charlotte clacked away at the keyboard. Up popped a screen with *"The Lakeside Line"* emblazoned across the top in bold, nautical-blue letters on a silver-gray background. A red lure on a fishing line arched across the page, creating a wave for the letters to float upon.

"Nice."

"Kate set everything up for me. It's not much, but I'm not as savvy with this stuff as you young people. I often forget to update it."

Charlotte tapped through the four static web pages, which included a short history of the paper, info regarding deadlines, a patron subscription form, and a contact page. At the bottom of one of the pages was a button titled "Sutton Stories." Charlotte assumed it was her father's sports articles. Of course, he'd want to give his readers a glimpse of his limelight moments—Chuck the Narcissist at his best.

Charlotte scrolled back to the homepage. "Maybe expand the website and dump your headline story and a community calendar on here after every issue. Once a new issue comes out, you could include the previous week's back issue online. If you gave people a reason to come to the site, advertisers might be interested in buying space on your home page."

"Really?"

"It wouldn't take that much time. I could set it up for you, if you want. And I'm pretty sure Kate could handle the updates."

"You'd do that for me?"

"Sure. It's what I do. I help businesses with stuff like this—content writing, social media posts, whatever the agency needs me to do."

"Well, thanks. I'd appreciate that." Chuck leaned back in his chair, suddenly spent. "I can't keep up with the technology anymore. I'm getting too old for this... forgetting about the lack of memory, for a moment."

Charlotte let loose a bark of laughter.

Chuck frowned.

"Forgetting the lack of memory?" Charlotte's eyes locked on his, so like her own. "Sorry. That was rude of me."

"Oh." Chuck shrugged. "Well, if we can't see the humor in forgetting, what's the point? Right, kid?"

They both smiled.

Glancing at his notes, Chuck honed in on the lone pink piece of paper in the top right corner of the table. He read it and crossed to the filing cabinet, opened the bottom drawer, and pulled out a white envelope. "CHARLIE" was written on the outside.

Chuck motioned to the envelope. "Can we please try again?"

"Try what?" Charlotte said warily.

"To talk about the Power of Attorney. I've completed the paperwork. It's all in here. Everything's been notarized on my end. There's going to come a time when I can't remember. You'll be in charge, Charlie. You'll have to remember for me."

He returned to the table and laid the envelope across Charlotte's thighs. She refused to look at the thing—the weight of the world in her lap.

A weight she had no interest in taking on.

"No." As if it were a game of "hot potato," Charlotte tossed the envelope onto the table. It slid, uprooting a couple of notes in the process, and almost went off the edge. Chuck snapped it up before it could drop. He flipped the envelope to show the name "CHARLIE" face up and gave his daughter a look.

"Come on. This isn't easy for me. Do you think I like having to rely on notes to get through my day? Do you think I like asking other people to manage my affairs? I have to plan for what's ahead."

"I get it," Charlotte said. "But I've wanted to be free from small-town Ohio most of my life. Why would I allow myself to be sucked back in again? You're asking too much. I can't deal with this. I don't want the responsibility."

"It's your choice. I can't make you."

"No. No, you can't. Not anymore." Charlotte noted the clock above her father's head. "It's almost time for your appointment."

"What?"

"Your neurology appointment at 10 o'clock."

"Neurology appointments are for sissies."

"Sure, Chuck."

15

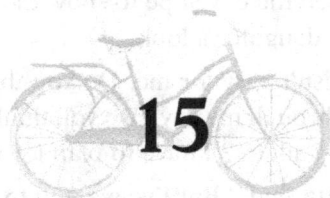

Chuck rode in silence, staring out the window at the passing cars. The Jenson & Bentley Medical Center office, located in Marblehead and housed in an old, sandstone building, sported a painted red-and-white-striped pole at the entrance—a holdover from the previous barber tenant. The neurology doctor apparently saw no irony in presenting the storefront to its patients as anything other than a medical facility.

"Messing with the mind, when the mind is already a mess," Charlotte muttered, pulling into a parking spot.

"What?"

"Nothing. Just internal commentary on your medical community. Maybe we could do lunch at Quarters, if it's open by the time we're done," Charlotte said. "It was always my favorite."

Chuck nodded. "I'd like that. They still make a mean piece of pie."

Chuck signed in, and they both took a seat in the waiting room reeking of vanilla air freshener and antiseptic. A quarter of an hour later, they were taken to a room, and the nurse, Amanda something, took Chuck's vitals and had him roll up a sleeve.

"Let's see if we can find a vein here, Mr. Sutton. You fasted, right?"

"Yes."

"I didn't know you needed to fast," Charlotte said.

"We're checking his thyroid and vitamin B12 levels," the nurse said. "He had us program the reminder into his phone before he left the last appointment."

Charlotte nodded. "Smart."

Chuck grimaced. "Play smarter, not harder, I always say. I can't wait too long to write anything down."

The nurse finished drawing blood and left the room. Above the desk was a print of the human brain, and on the desk sat a model to scale, complete with removable, multicolored sections. Chuck pulled out a portion and held it up to the light, turning it left and right.

"I did research on Alzheimer's, a long time ago. It was for a feature during Alzheimer's Awareness Month." Chuck pointed to the brain piece in his hand. "They say it's all about the neurons and when they stop functioning. The parts of the brain involving memory go first—the entorhinal cortex and hippocampus. How is it that I can remember a bunch of medical jargon I learned many years back, but don't know where I mislaid my keys this morning?"

"I forget where I put my keys, too, Chuck."

"Really?" Charlotte's father juggled the brain section back and forth in his hands, like a misshaped baseball, before fitting it neatly back into the hole. "Do you ever find them in the refrigerator?"

"No."

"It's a thing," Chuck said softly.

This is your brain. This is your brain on Alzheimer's.

"Why don't we talk about something else, while we're waiting?"

"Okay." Chuck leaned back in his chair, an ankle resting on a knee. "How is your writing going, Charlie? Anything new in *The Boston Globe*?"

"How'd you know about that?"

"Your mom and I don't hate each other as much as you think. In fact, we're better friends now than when we were married. She keeps me in the loop, more or less. I usually get the link to anything with your name on it, about a minute after you send it to her."

"Huh." Charlotte found it hard to reconcile her childhood memories of the fights, the absences, and the hurt she and her mother experienced before, during, and after the divorce. Was this the new reality? Her parents happily exchanging emails about her, like cooks exchanging recipes?

"You're a good writer, kid. I really enjoyed your piece about growing up with Lake Erie in your front yard."

"Yeah, well, the lake and I have always had a... good thing." Charlotte shrugged. "I missed it. That's what I missed most."

A range of emotions flitted across Chuck's face. "I thought you wanted to live in the big city? Pittsburgh isn't doing it for you?"

"Sure. I like it there well enough. It's just different, I guess. I like watching the motorboats on the Allegheny River, but it isn't Lake Erie. It doesn't have her personality. And there really isn't anywhere close to go sailing."

Chuck leaned over and took Charlotte's hand. He turned it over, palm side up.

"No calluses, huh? I can remember you were a mess at the end of every summer, from gripping the lines."

Charlotte pulled her hand into her lap. "I never liked wearing gloves."

"You were a great little sailor. Took to it like a duck to water."

"We both know that isn't true."

"But you loved it?"

"Yes, and that's all that really mattered... to me."

Silence filled the gap between them.

"Any boyfriends in Pittsburgh that matter to you?"

Charlotte sighed. "Not really."

118

"Just trying to keep up."

"I dated a guy from work for a while, but it's over. At least for me. Elliot is a little harder to convince."

"I see."

There was a light tap on the door.

"Come in," Chuck said.

A smallish woman entered. Her hair was a beehive of worry, unruly tight gray curls poking out from a bun at the base of her neck.

"Good morning," she said. "How are we doing today?"

Chuck smiled. "You look lovely as always, Nola."

A bright spot of red leapt to the doctor's cheeks. "Always the silver tongue. I wasn't asking about me, Chuck, but thank you." She thrust her birdlike hand toward Charlotte. "Dr. Nola Jenson. You must be Charlie."

Charlotte threw her father a look. "Charlotte. His only daughter. That I know of."

"I've heard so much about you."

"Really?"

The doctor nodded. "Your dad and I played in a euchre league for the past several winters. He's quite the card shark."

"Used to be. Nola was the one that first picked up on what was going on with me," Chuck said.

"Unfortunately, or fortunately, if you'd rather, I do have a knack for noticing these things," Dr. Jenson said. "Chuck started forgetting when it was his turn, what the trump suit was, and so on. I asked him to come in to chat about six months ago."

"*Six* months?" Charlotte shook her head. "This has been going on that long? Why didn't anyone tell me sooner?"

"You didn't want to come back home," Chuck said. "And I didn't want to bother you until we knew more."

Charlotte looked everywhere but into Dr. Jenson's eyes. "So, what's the story? Where are you with the diagnosis?"

"Straight to the point. I like that." The doctor pulled a folder from the file holder hanging on the door.

"I told you she's a pretty good kid," Chuck said.

I'm a grown-assed adult. You barely know me.

"Smart, too," Chuck added.

Dr. Jenson tapped the folder. "Since I'd already been observing your father, we bypassed his primary care physician. I've done all the initial testing, including the physical exam and some bloodwork to rule out other medical issues. I've still got a few things up my sleeve, but your father does show symptoms of early-onset Alzheimer's disease. He's young, but this is not unheard of."

"I'd read that," Charlotte said.

"I will give you some more educational information before you go," the doctor said. "There are medications that may slow down the progression of the disease."

Chuck motioned to the paper-clad examination table. "Shall I assume the position?"

"No need." Dr. Jenson picked up a pen. "We're just doing the verbal tests today." She turned toward Charlotte. "Jake came with your dad to the last appointment, but from now on, a family member must accompany him. Those who see him daily need to let me know any changes since the last appointment. Chuck can only tell me what he remembers. He may not be the most reliable source of information, as we move forward."

"Oh," Charlotte said.

"We'll also need to schedule a PET scan—Positron Emission Tomography. It may help detect plaques in the brain. I've already run a CT scan and MRI. No signs of tumors, stroke, or anything else that might cause similar dementia symptoms."

Charlotte winced. Franco Bellimer was right. She *would* need to come up from Pittsburgh if she wanted to avoid Adam having to tag along to Chuck's future appointments. Her gaze slid to Chuck. His eyes were closed, his lips clenched.

"Can we get this over with?" Chuck muttered.

Dr. Jenson nodded. "Absolutely. Let's start with the obvious. What is your full name?"

"Charles Adam Sutton."

"Chuck, at the end of this test, I will ask you questions about the following short story. Lily jogged to the sea and discovered five seagulls on a post. She picked up a dozen shells for her niece, Abigail. Got that?"

"Sure."

"Let's continue. How old are you?"

"55."

"55 plus 12 equals what?"

"I'm sorry?"

"55 plus 12 equals?"

"67."

"Where was Charlotte born?"

"Port Clinton, Ohio."

"What is her middle name?"

Chuck paused. "Elise."

Charlotte leaned forward. "No—"

Dr. Jenson shook her head at Charlotte.

"Elise is my ex-wife," Chuck said. "We were going to call her 'Charlotte Elise Sutton' but ended up going with 'Anne,' after my mother."

Dr. Jenson looked at Charlotte. She nodded.

"Good, Chuck," the doctor said. "How many days are there in a week?"

"Not enough. There are seven days in a week."

"Very good." Dr. Jenson handed Chuck her pen and a blank piece of paper. "Please draw a clock face."

Chuck did so, though his numbers didn't quite fit properly on the circle. The first three-quarters of the numbers jumbled, willy-nilly, against each other, the "9" resting at the normal "7" spot. The final section of the pie remained blank.

"I'm not much of an artist," Chuck said, letting the pen roll from his fingers.

"That's okay." Dr. Jenson made a mark in her folder. "Can you count backwards from 100 by fives?" Chuck did so, miscalculating only once. Dr. Jenson made another note.

The doctor put Chuck through several more benchmark tests, all the while making notes. A pressure built in Charlotte's chest every time the pen met paper. How Chuck could take it with such easy calm—always the easy calm—she couldn't grasp.

"Do you remember what I said you'd need to recall at the end of the test?"

"Sorry?"

"I told you a short story about a woman. Do you remember anything about that?"

"Oh. Yes, her name was Lily, like the flower. She went to the shore."

"Which shore?"

Charlotte held her breath.

"Lake Erie?"

It was the ocean, Chuck. She went to the sea.

"Can you remember what she found at the shore?"

"Waves? And seagulls."

"How many? Was it five, 55, or a dozen?"

"I don't remember. 55?"

Five. Five, Chuck. You're 55 years old.

"Lily picked up shells for someone," Dr. Jenson said. "Do you recall who?"

"Her niece."

Good, Chuck.

"What was her niece's name?"

Charlotte glanced down at her father's hands. Clenched into fists on his knees, they'd lost their color but for the blue vein snaking across the back of his right fist. "Abby? Gail. Her name was Gail."

Abigail. Lily jogged to the sea and discovered five seagulls on a post. She picked up a dozen shells for her niece, Abigail.

Charlotte reached out and put her hand over her father's. His skin was dry and leathery, soft to the touch. Chuck slowly relaxed beneath her palm and allowed his fingers to cup his knee.

"You did great, Dad," Charlotte murmured.

A faint smile flickered on Chuck's lips.

It was the first time she'd called her father "Dad" in 10 years, maybe longer.

Definitely longer.

Charlotte wasn't sure exactly how she felt about it.

"Thanks, Charlie." Chuck's hand turned in hers, and he gave her fingers a squeeze. He slumped back in his chair.

16

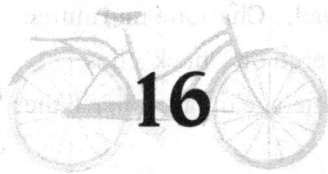

Gripping the wheel, Charlotte peered through the window. She breathed in, breathed out. Finally, she punched the ignition button and glanced at Chuck sitting beside her.

"Well, that sucked. Are you okay?"

He slumped against the door and closed his eyes. "Yeah. Just tired. Every appointment makes me tired. It's like my brain gets a workout."

Charlotte buckled her seatbelt. "It felt like we were in there for days."

The appointment had taken just under an hour. How did her father do it?

"You mind if we stop by The Clip Joint before getting lunch? I want to talk to Sammy again before I leave this afternoon. He can't stay mad at me forever. I won't let him."

"Sure. Fine."

Charlotte reversed out of her parking spot. "Don't forget your seatbelt."

"Right." Chuck fumbled for the strap and pulled it across his waist.

The car rolled past the post office and a boarded-up pastry shop. A loud pinging prompted Charlotte to look down. Her father still held the seatbelt near his left hip.

"Your seatbelt." With only one eye on the road, she reached down and guided his hand. The pinging stopped.

"Dammit. Sorry," Chuck said.

"No worries." Charlotte pulled into a spot in front of The Clip Joint. "You can stay in the car and rest. I'll just be a minute. Promise."

"Jesus, Charlie. I'm fine. I'm not kicking the bucket today, for shit's sake." Chuck's voice rose. "Quit treating me like a damn toddler."

What the hell? Charlotte bristled. Chuck sounded like her potty-mouth mother in that moment. She could never remember him cursing at anyone, not even Elise.

"Sorry, kid." Chuck groaned and rammed his shoulder into the passenger's side door. He stepped onto the sidewalk.

Charlotte scrambled to do the same. "It's fine."

"I didn't mean to snap," Chuck said. "Just tired, is all. Those appointments always make me look like a fool."

"You didn't look like a fool."

"Sure, I did." Chuck shrugged. "Never mind. I'm stopping in Stanner's Hardware for a moment. Need some lightbulbs."

"You don't want to come in and say 'hi' to Sammy?" Charlotte motioned to the salon.

"No. You have your moment with him, Charlie. Take your time. If I get done first, I'll pop my head in. His mom has a crush on me."

"How in the heck would you know that?"

Chuck offered a weak smile. "A man always knows."

"Whatever." Charlotte rolled her eyes. At least he was acting a little more like himself.

Barely.

"If you're sure? See you in a few minutes, then, and we'll walk to Quarters for lunch."

"Right." Chuck shuffled down the sidewalk. He waved in greeting to a man walking in the other direction, and the gentleman, about Chuck's age, stopped and grasped his hand.

Her father should have been a politician. Charlotte turned, hopped over the welcome mat, and set the bells tinkling. Mrs. Macon looked up from the register, and a smile spread across her face.

"Charlotte, you came back."

"Of course, Mama. I told you I would. Sammy in?" Charlotte snagged a shortbread cookie from the tray on the counter.

"I'm afraid not, sweet girl. You just missed him. He only had one appointment this morning, so he went to buy supplies. Are you going to make up with my boy?"

"I want to try." Charlotte frowned. It would be wrong to disappear again, without fixing things with Sammy—really, really wrong.

"Can you do me a favor, Mama?"

"Anything."

Charlotte fished in her pocket and pulled out her phone.

"Can you give me his number?"

"Oh, Charlotte, I don't know—"

"Please, Mama, it's important. I need to make this right."

Mama tilted her head. "You certainly do." She motioned to Charlotte's phone.

"Thanks, Mama."

* * * * *

Charlotte stood by the hood of her car and stared down at her phone.

Dude, call me ASAP—

Nope.

Charlotte erased the text message.

Pls call—

She erased that one, too.

Charlotte glanced toward The Clip Joint. He was angry, and she had no idea how to fix it. Sighing, she finally settled on the obvious.

Sorry—

Charlotte pressed send. It would have to do.

Pushing the thought to the back of her mind, she walked several doors down to Stanner's Hardware. When she stepped through the door, Jim Stanner looked up from the cash register and smiled with his whole ruddy face.

"Charlie Sutton, well aren't you a beautiful sight? I heard you'd come back."

"I bet." Charlotte blinked. "Wow, Jim, you look great."

Jim's face deepened a shade. "Gosh, thanks."

A year behind Charlotte in school, the youngest son of the Stanner's Hardware family had always been one of the shortest, least physically fit guys in his class. He'd grown about a foot and, apparently, been on a self-improvement kick since graduation.

"I started doing 5Ks three years ago," Jim said, flexing a bicep. "Made some changes to my diet. Started taking yoga classes. So, you've been living in Steelers Country?"

"Yep. Been in Pittsburgh since high school. I went to Carnegie Mellon." Charlotte glanced past Jim. She had a view of just about every aisle the length of the small store, and it appeared she was the only potential customer.

"Well, welcome home," Jim said. "How about we catch a football game at the tavern some Sunday and catch up? My treat."

Charlotte's attention snapped back to the man in front of her.

"We'll have to pick a date," Jim said. "I'd like to get together. I'd like that a *whole* lot, Charlie. Sure would."

A date? Charlotte shook her head. "Thanks, but I'm actually going back this afternoon. I'm just here dealing with some family stuff. So, um, is Chuck in the back talking to your dad? I thought he was buying lightbulbs."

Jim's broad shoulders slumped. "Chuck? No, I haven't seen him."

Charlotte sucked in a breath. "Really? Would you mind checking for me?"

"Sure thing. Give me a sec."

Jim disappeared into the back room.

Charlotte scanned the aisles again. The shelves held only the most essential of tools and home supplies alongside custom lake t-shirts and sunscreen. Marblehead commerce had usually existed on two realms. Businesses were either operated by the same family for decades, like Stanner's Hardware, or they cycled through new ownership every few years, as wannabe seasonal shopkeepers failed or succeeded at making a living doing most of their business in the three hottest tourism months of the year. The Stanners had figured out the sweet spot between the homeowners' needs and the tourists' wants.

Jim returned, followed by his father. About 100 pounds heavier than his son, Randy Stanner clutched a wooden walking stick with a carving of a bald eagle gracing the top. Acne scars branched across his cheeks and down his neck.

"Charlie Sutton." Randy's voice boomed, ricocheting off the high, tin ceilings of the old building. "Well, by gosh. Great to see you. You're all grown up."

Charlotte smiled. "Hey, Mr. Stanner. Yeah, it's been ten years. Has Chuck been in?"

"Sorry, not for a couple of months. I've called a few times to let him know we need his signature on the annual contract to set up his heating and cooling maintenance for the cottage. Can you sign off on it for me? Save me some postage."

"Oh." Charlotte frowned. "Um, sure."

"Gotta be here somewhere." Randy rifled through a pile of file folders, and Charlotte's mind ticked off the possibilities. Had Chuck gone back to the car? She glanced toward the window. She couldn't see her vehicle from the shop.

Randy pulled a folder from the middle and laid a contract on the counter. He offered Charlotte a pen with a plastic daisy taped to its end, one from a bouquet of them in a coffee can by the register.

"I heard your dad is having some health issues. Anything we can do to help?"

Charlotte barely looked at what she was signing. She glanced again toward the window.

"Yeah, I don't know yet, exactly. We just came from the doctor's office."

Randy came around the counter and laid a beefy hand on Charlotte's shoulder, his grasp gentle. "He's in our prayers. You know that, right?" Randy offered a business card from the counter. "Take this and don't hesitate to call me or Jimmy. We're here for you, if you need anything at all."

"Thank you. I appreciate that." Charlotte accepted the card and stuffed it in her back pocket. A shiver ran up her spine as she began slowly backing toward the door. She missed the warmth of old Stanner's hand. "I've... I've got to go find Chuck."

"Great to see you again," Randy said. "Don't be such a stranger."

"Take care you don't wear too much black and gold around here," Jim said. "You were born a Dawg. Woof. Woof. Woof."

"Sure." With a sweaty palm, Charlotte gripped the doorknob and bolted from the building. Maybe she'd misunderstood Chuck. Maybe he'd misunderstood her. She fumbled for her phone and scrolled to her contacts.

No. It was pointless.

She'd wiped his cell number from her contact list long ago. And she didn't have Adam's. There was no way to reach either of them.

Had he gone to lunch? Marblehead Captain's Quarters, a place in business in the same location as long as she could remember and dubbed "Quarters" by the locals, sat in the distance several blocks east. Charlotte hurried past the closed library and a soap shop. Her heart beating faster with every step, she ran past the ferry dock and a strip of abandoned storefronts. She poked her head into a gallery and two gift stores, but saw no sign of her father and didn't recognize any other store owners.

She crossed the street and approached the entrance to Quarters.

Through the window, she saw her father sitting at the bar with a beer in front of him. Relief swept through her, immediately followed by a flush of irritation. Chuck lifted the drink, his eyes trained on the television above him. It was tuned to a sports channel.

Figures. Charlotte took a deep breath and entered. "I've been looking for you everywhere." She threw her coat on the back of the chair next to Chuck's. "Seriously, Chuck, how come you didn't go into Stanner's?"

Chuck turned. "I'm sorry? Do I—"

"I thought we were meeting there." Plopping her bag on the bar, Charlotte began rummaging for her phone. "Before I head back to Pittsburgh, I've got to put your number in my contacts. I couldn't find you. You scared the crap out of me."

"I didn't mean... what?"

Charlotte stopped fidgeting long enough to register the confusion in her father's eyes. A chill raced up her spine, making her twitch.

Oh, no.

"Who are—"

Please. Please. Please, no.

"Oh, Dad. I'm so sorry," Charlotte whispered. Bile rose in her throat. She swallowed and carefully laid a hand on her father's forearm.

"It's me, Dad. Charlie. Your daughter. Care to share a piece of peanut butter pie?"

17

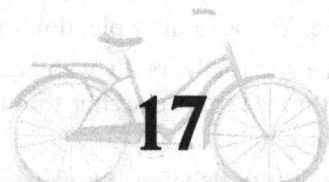

ELEMENTARY SCHOOL

Nine-year-old Charlotte rubbed her aching legs—limp, like carrots left too long in the refrigerator. Her feet ached, and the thick socks had bunched during the game. She was totally sure she had a blister on her left heel. She picked hardened flecks of mud off her thighs and dropped the offending proof of her latest athletic failure onto the backseat floor mat.

Soccer sucks.

Sucks. Sucks. Sucks.

"You did pretty well out there, Charlie. Glad I could make it for the second half," her father said from the driver's seat. "You've just got to pay attention to what's going on around you. Watch what's happening on the field. You're smart and a head taller than most of them. Refuse to lose, kid. Use your height to your advantage."

"Sure, Dad."

Charlotte slumped down in her seat and picked another hardened ball from her knee. She held it up to inspect it and, aiming carefully, flicked it at the back of her father's head. Per usual, her eye-hand coordination failed her. It struck a bit too low, bouncing off the seat and back into Charlotte's lap. She brushed it off onto the floor to join its muddy brothers and sisters.

"If you fall down, you've got to pick yourself right back up and have another go at it. Hard work beats talent when talent doesn't work hard. Soccer is the ticket, Charlie. Much better fit than softball. It's all about being the smartest kid on the field."

"Sure, Dad."

"You did great, honey," Mom said, her voice higher than normal. "What your father meant to say is that we love you, no matter what. You did your best, and that's all that matters. Next stop, Quarters and peanut butter pie. You love their pie, don't you, Charlotte?"

Mom sounded like she really, really wanted to let fly one of her colorful words. She threw a smile over her shoulder, but the look on her face was, in a word, tight.

Tight? Tense? Charlotte debated the word choice. In language arts class, her teacher would probably say Mom was tense.

What a boring word. Tense.

Charlotte pulled her journal from her soccer bag and jotted down a note to look up synonyms for tense. There had to be something less boring.

Chuck pulled the sedan into the restaurant parking lot and cut the engine.

"Leave your journal in the car, honey," Mom said. "Let's go eat."

Charlotte followed her parents into Marblehead Captain's Quarters. In this one case, she kind of liked that everyone had nicknamed it Quarters. Marblehead Captain's Quarters was a mouthful and brought to mind a somewhat disturbing mental image of her father's old multi-colored marbles—aggies and bumblebees and cat's eyes—spewing out his mouth like gumballs with every quarter placed in his ear.

Quarters was a better name. Short. To the point.

Charlotte liked short and to the point.

I wish I were short.

While they waited to be seated, Chuck raised his hand to the Kim family in the corner. Jenny Kim, also dressed in soccer gear, plunged her fingers into a basket of fries.

"Come this way," the waitress said.

Charlotte followed her parents to a table next to the Kims.

"Wow." Chuck slid into his chair. "Jenny, you sure tore up the field today. You were all over the place, weren't you, kid? That score late in the second half was fantastic. How many points did you end up with?"

"Thanks, Mr. Sutton." A glob of ketchup hung from Jenny's lower lip. "Three goals."

"Napkin, sweetie," Mrs. Kim whispered.

Chuck grabbed some napkins from the dispenser and handed them over. "How long have you played soccer?"

"Since she was five," Mr. Kim said. "We had her in gymnastics before that."

Jenny grinned. "I like soccer way better. I can get dirty."

"Is soccer your favorite sport?" Chuck said.

"Sure, but I love softball, too. And basketball and swimming and maybe someday I'll try hockey."

"A girl after my own heart."

Charlotte fidgeted with her silverware wrapped in a paper napkin. The spinning knife struck her water glass with a loud clang, and her mother placed a hand over hers. The silverware fell silent.

"Did you have fun at soccer today, Charlotte?" Mr. Kim said.

Charlotte's stomach clenched. "Sure?"

"That was your first game, right?" Mr. Kim smiled. "It just takes practice. You'll get the hang of it."

"Uh-huh." Feeling a burning behind her eyelids, Charlotte quickly got up from her chair. "Excuse me. I'm going to wash my hands. Mom, can you please order me a burger and lemonade?"

"Of course, honey."

Charlotte hurried to the bathroom. She rushed into the first open stall and closed the door. Tears ran in silent rivulets down her cheeks. The flush of the toilet in the next stall hid her gulp for air.

Soccer sucks. Sucks. Sucks. Sucks.

Charlotte rolled the itchy, knee-length soccer socks down to her ankles and took deep breaths. The water at the sink took forever to shut off. Finally, the bathroom door thumped shut.

"Thank God." Charlotte ran her fingernails up and down her bare legs, scratching red welts into the skin, but the pain did nothing to calm her. She gulped more breaths.

"Charlotte?"

Charlotte stilled at the sound of Jenny's voice.

"You in here?"

"Upset stomach. I'll be out in a minute."

"All right."

Water trickled at the sink, and the door slammed a second time. Leaving her stall, Charlotte washed her face and patted her blotchy eyes with a paper towel soaked in cold water. She undid the long braid hanging over one shoulder and allowed her mass of wavy hair to fall forward, a black curtain to help hide most everything. She would never be Jenny. Not even close.

Charlotte returned to the table. Jenny glanced up, meeting her eyes and turning away. Mom said nothing. Chuck continued his conversation with Mr. Kim about the intricacies of various sports, which Cleveland team had the better chance of a winning season, and what writing he was doing at the moment. He entertained them with his most recent trip to New York City to accept a sports award.

Charlotte picked at her food.

"*Smokin' Smokey Joe* took a long time to research," Chuck said, "but the press has been very kind. Great reviews, particularly since the award list came out. I've been so busy, I'm barely home."

"Aren't you hungry, sweetie?" Mom placed her hand on Charlotte's knee.

Charlotte shrugged and buried her barely touched burger beneath her napkin. The waitress came back and asked if they wanted dessert, and her mother ordered a piece of peanut butter pie to go.

When they stood to leave, Chuck shook Mr. Kim's hand and patted Jenny on the shoulder as he passed.

"Great job on the field today, kid."

"Thanks, Mr. Sutton," Jenny said.

Charlotte hugged herself and trailed behind her parents and out the door.

Mom glanced over her shoulder. She looked tense again.

"It's okay, sweetie."

Tense. What a boring word.

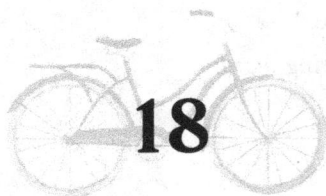

18

Charlotte,

So sorry to hear about your father. Please take all the time you need. I'll send your projects through, and when you're back after Thanksgiving, let's chat about a possible uptick in your responsibilities. We're taking on a new client in the spring, and they've requested a dedicated writer to work with their marketing team. You'd be a good fit, and it would be full-time. Keep us posted about your return date. —T

*   *   *   *   *

After Chuck's neurology appointment and his incident in Marblehead, Charlotte had contacted the ad agency and requested several weeks to get her father's affairs in order. She re-read the email from her boss. Tania had accommodated her and even hinted at a promotion. The full-time writing gig would provide a steady income, something Charlotte had been working hard toward.

It would be a stepping stone—a placeholder on her resume leading to something bigger and better. Though she was good at it, the advertising materials she wrote for clients were too one-sided. She never got to research and form her own opinion, or write both sides of the story like her father did with the newspaper. She envied him that. In advertising, only the opinion of the client mattered. She was more a salesman than a writer. But that was the point, wasn't it? She was being paid to sell whatever product she was being paid to sell.

Shaking off the inkling she was missing something, Charlotte powered down her computer and sent a quick text to Elliot.

Busy with Dad. Back after Turkey Day. Hug furry guy—

He'd been buzzing her non-stop since she'd arrived. She *really* never should have taken Alfredo for a walk.

Charlotte followed up the Elliot text with another one to Sammy.

Sorry Sorry Sorry Sorry—

He hadn't responded to her last three texts, but he'd have to give in eventually.

Pressing "send," she stared down at her blank phone screen, wishing she didn't have to do what she had to do next.

Charlotte held the phone to her ear, her eyes glazing over with each ring.

Mom is going to have a cow.

Maybe she wouldn't pick up. Charlotte had messaged Elise but received no response back. Perhaps, she was off to the southern coast of Rome with Husband #2. Charlotte had gotten the sense Antonio was more proud than jealous of the attention his sassy, middle-aged American wife had received from Italian men of all ages since their move to Ostia.

Elise answered suddenly with a tinkle of laughter. "Ciao bella. How's the 'Burgh, my love? Getting cold? You should come visit."

"Morning, Mom."

"It's afternoon, here, sweetie. We're six hours ahead."

"Oh, right. How's Antonio?"

"Simply perfect. He's a hot-blooded Italian. He loves me. I am his everything."

Her mother was happier than Charlotte had ever known her to be, although Elise had snapped up, and just as quickly discarded, a number of male friends since Chuck. She'd taken the trip down the aisle with Antonio, but Charlotte didn't have a lot of faith the pairing would, ultimately, fare much better.

"So, what's the word, sweetie?"

Charlotte hesitated. "Dad's having some health issues."

Silence on the other end. Too long.

"Mom?"

There was a heavy sigh.

"Chuck is absolutely fine," Elise said. "That asshat is just looking for sympathy. You know, I told him to grow himself a pair and go visit you in Pittsburgh, instead of constantly flaking out. For *years* the idiot didn't listen to me, and now he's pulling this bullshit to get your attention? Really, Charlotte, it's ridiculous. What he owes you is an apology. Ignore him."

A familiar ache flooded Charlotte's stomach.

"What do you mean, flaking out?"

"He's still calling from time to time and hanging up, isn't he?"

"What?"

"He had his chance to be a father to you, and he blew it. That's on him. Suck it up, buttercup, is what I told him. You've got to just talk to Charlotte. That's all she wants, but, oh, no. He's just too much of a shitfest to get the job done."

A rush of anger pulled Charlotte to her feet and, for the first time, she felt like she needed to defend her father. Elise could be vicious.

"He may not have much longer to try, Mom. He's really sick. I'm in Ohio right now, and I'm staying for a few weeks, so I can take him to his next doctor's appointment."

"Doctor's appointment?"

"A neurologist. Dr. Nolan says he probably has Alzheimer's. I thought you'd want to know."

Her mother gasped.

"One second, honey."

Elise blew her nose, ferociously, in the background. She was soon back on the line.

"You okay, Mom?"

"Just allergies." Elise's voice had lost its swagger. "You're sure? About your dad?"

"I went with him this week." Charlotte recapped the neurology appointment and explained what she'd learned after looking over the materials and notes from the doctor. "It's serious, Mom. The doctor thinks he's been compensating for his memory loss for a long time. He's much farther along than anyone knew, and he's getting worse. He has really good days, like nothing's wrong. But other days—

"But, Charlotte, I don't understand. How long does he have—"

"We... we don't know," Charlotte said. "It could be a few years or a decade. The disease is just that unpredictable, Mom. Even if Dr. Nolan's meds help stall the symptoms, there's no cure."

"Oh, sweetie." Elise's voice dipped. "I'm so sorry. Really. Do you need me to come home? That poor son of a bitch. Is Chuck in any pain?"

"He's okay." Charlotte hesitated. "At least for now." It surprised her that her mother would offer. After her parents split, Elise had made a sport of bitching about Chuck, and Charlotte couldn't remember her having anything kind to say about him since. She had learned to tune it out, mostly.

"Let me know if you need me. He's a jackass, but he's *our* jackass, and he *is* your father."

"Thanks, Mom. There's, um, something else I need to talk to you about."

The pause on the other end stretched on forever. Charlotte decided to let it.

"What would that be, honey?" Elise said finally.

"What do you think?"

"Aaaaah. Chuck finally let the bastard skeleton out of the closet, did he?"

"Mom! That's a horrible thing to say. It's not his fault."

"Hell it isn't. Good-time Charlie couldn't keep it in his pants."

Charlotte winced. "I meant Adam. It's not *Adam's* fault."

"You're right, sweetie. Not very Christian of me, but Chuck always brings out my Satan side. Of course, it isn't that boy's fault, but it's about damned time Chuck took responsibility for screwing that awful woman."

"Why didn't you tell me I have a brother?"

"What's done is done."

"Hardly. You love having something to hold over Dad. I would have expected you to take out an ad in *The Lakeside Line* about this one. Why didn't you say something?"

Silence.

"Mom?"

A heavy sigh filtered through the line. "It wasn't my place to tell you. Let's just say your dad and I were equally to blame for the divorce. We recognize that now. I don't want to rehash everything. When I found out he'd found himself a little toy in Cleveland, I was pissed. I may have acted like a child about the whole thing. Goose. Gander. I got him back."

"What?" The ache in Charlotte's stomach intensified.

"Now, sweetie, calm down—"

"You cheated, too? With Antonio? How could you?"

"No, no." Elise brushed it off. "Not Antonio. Someone else... long before Antonio. Someone I met at a bar. It was nothing, sweetie. Just me getting back at your daddy."

"Unbelievable." Charlotte's voice dropped. "Simply unbelievable. You're as bad as he is. Worse, even. At least he did it with a friend."

"Come now, Charlotte. Don't be like that. Shit, child, we're not perfect."

"Yeah, I'd say not."

"You're not perfect either. Nobody is. We're *human*. We make mistakes and we do stupid shit. That's what humans do."

"I just would have expected—"

"Better?" Elise asked. "We *should* have done better, but we didn't. You've always had such high expectations of everyone. You can't even live up to the expectations you set for *yourself*, sweetie. Lighten up already. We didn't love each other anymore. We screwed someone else. We got a divorce. That's it. What's past is past."

Charlotte dropped her head into her hands, barely able to keep the phone pressed to her ear. How could her mother speak so lightly of it? Both her parents had cheated. Did that somehow cancel out each other's transgression? Make them both or neither to blame?

"What a mess."

"Don't be too hard on us," Elise said. "What's important is that your dad and I still love *you*, even if we don't love each other. We always have, and we always will. We love you so very much, baby."

"Love you, too, Mom," Charlotte mumbled.

Elise's Pomeranian yipped in the background.

"Antonio is home. I've got to go now. You take care of Chuck, and call me if you need me." Charlotte could hear the slight hitch in her mother's voice. "And tell the ass... tell your father I said 'hello.' He got pretty decent at emailing me from time to time, and I wondered why I hadn't heard from him lately. Guess it was the Alzheimer's. I've been sending him links to all your articles." Another muffled sniffle. "He's so proud of you." The barking intensified. "Addio, sweetie."

The line went dead.

Charlotte stared down at her phone. It was too much.

She plucked her shoes from the floor and padded down the stairs. The cottage was empty. Adam was at school and Chuck already at

141

the office. She grabbed her coat and had just gotten in her car when Jake strolled around the corner of the house. Sydney trailed after him, barking for all she was worth.

Like the time before, if Charlotte just pilfered the rocker and ran away, she could forget this ever happened. She rested her head briefly on the wheel then rolled down the window.

"Hey, Jake."

"I just stopped by to see how things are going."

"Great." Charlotte sought the calm of his blue eyes. What she found was worry.

Jake crossed his arms. "Great, huh? So, what are you doing?"

"Nothing drastic, if that's what you're thinking. Though I'm tempted." Charlotte gave him a meager smile. "Just going for a ride around the peninsula. I need to think some things through. Would you check on my dad at the office? I might be gone a while."

"Sure. Whatever you need."

"Can you let him know I probably won't be home for dinner? Or tell Bea, since he might not remember?"

"Roger. Got it."

"Thanks."

"Good luck, Charlotte." Jake patted the hood of the car, and she backed out of the drive.

How many times would she regret having come home in the first place?

19

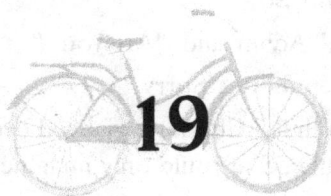

Charlotte returned to the cottage later that afternoon. Her father was not yet home. She peered out the screen door to the front porch and found Adam reading in her favorite rocker.

Here goes nothing.

The door shut behind Charlotte with a muffled thud.

"Hey."

Adam looked up from the book—a blank page—and immediately closed it. He clipped a pen on the front cover.

A journal? It was the same style as her father's journals and her own. Did Adam write? Charlotte crossed to the stairs and dropped down onto the top step. The wood slats beneath her sent a slight chill through her denims.

They needed to talk. To plan. It would not be an easy conversation. She expected to screw it up.

"Starting to get cold, huh?" she said.

"Yeah."

Charlotte shifted, leaning her shoulder against the porch post. It comforted her to feel the strength and stability of the structure that was Sutton's Choice, its foundation of more than 100 years as solid as the dock—as reliable as the waves to the north and, perhaps, Charlotte herself. What lay beneath her was certainly more stable than the air between brother and sister, thick with questions left unasked and unanswered. She was unsure if this fragile interaction could withstand the weight of her emotions.

Or Adam's, for that matter.

She took a breath. "So—"

"You came back," Adam said. "Are you—"

His question petered out. "Sorry."

"It's fine. You go first." Charlotte glanced over her shoulder and forced her lips to smile. She could only imagine how unnatural she looked.

Adam's eyes met hers. He shifted toward the lake. It was a southeast wind, sending spray up and over the dock and forming a slick slope upon contact. The temperature was expected to drop even further within the week, but it would be months before Lake Erie froze. Though it could be frigid during the winter, it was Charlotte's favorite Lakeside season—with the lake's personality at its fiercest and unadorned. Just the locals were lucky enough to play witness. She hadn't experienced it in a decade. Winters were something she remembered from her youth with a certain sense of pride.

"Are you staying?" Adam's voice was deep and nearly a whisper. "I'd just like to know, man."

Charlotte turned slightly toward him. Did he want her to stay or not? She suspected not.

"For now, I guess. I hadn't planned to, but maybe through Thanksgiving, just to get things in order. After that?" Charlotte shrugged. "I'm not sure."

"Why would you?"

She turned. "What do you mean?"

"Why would you stay?" Adam repeated. "You left Lakeside 10 years ago. You haven't been back since. When I called Dad earlier, he had no idea where you were. He thought you might have left *again*. Dude, you obviously don't like it here... or Dad."

"What do you know about what I like?" Charlotte kept her voice neutral, though it was a struggle. Regardless of what she liked or did not like, it was her decision to stay or go. It wasn't okay for some teenage boy to tell her how she felt.

"Dad didn't think you'd ever come back." Adam looked down at the journal in his hand, his thumb rubbing circles in the faded leather. "You could disappear again, whenever you want."

Not wrong. What kind of response was he looking for? They needed to get along and to talk through their options, slim as they were.

"You're just here because you have to be," Adam said.

Charlotte trained her gaze on the horizon. The sunset would not be worth much that evening, based on the cloud formation and years of watching hundreds of Lake Erie sunsets—each the same but different.

"You're right," she said finally. "And I feel like I have no choice but to stay. Not gonna lie, pretty much sucks not having any choice. If I stay, I'm right back where I started, and if I go, I'll feel guilty. I don't know how I feel about any of that. You probably don't want me here, and I get it. I'd feel the same if I were you. Chuck hasn't really given either of us much of a choice in this, though, has he?"

"Seriously?" Adam stood. "This isn't Dad's fault. Don't talk about choices. You left. That's on you, dude. I would never just up and leave. I'm lucky to even have a dad."

Charlotte shrugged. "Yes. You are. I've been living in Pittsburgh, dealing with life on my own without him or any communication from him. He might have been here for you, but that wasn't the case with me. I barely know him, and I'm still really struggling not to hate him for it. I *am* trying, Adam. It's not easy, and now I have all this responsibility dumped in my lap. I'm trying to deal with everything the best I can."

Adam rested his arms on the porch rail, his jaw thrust forward, gaze locked on the waters to their north. A ball hardened in Charlotte's chest. She'd said the wrong thing. Again. Her guilt was all wrapped up in that anger. Intertwined.

Guilt. Anger.

So much of both.

She'd always done what was expected to make others happy, then resented "them" when it didn't make *her* happy. Why did everyone else's concerns matter more than her own? This wasn't her fault, but it wasn't Adam's either. If anything, he was the least to blame for all of this.

Their current situation wasn't Chuck's fault either, though. Not really.

Alzheimer's was to blame. Simple genetics. It had taken away each of their choices, particularly Chuck's. Only Charlotte had the power to at least make some sense of the situation.

She knew it. Realized it.

Didn't like it.

"Look, I don't mean to be a bitch," Charlotte said. "I'm just being real with you. My relationship with Dad has never been great."

"That's your problem. It's got nothing to do with me."

Charlotte flinched. Adam's response reminded her, acutely, of her own childhood, when her mother would talk trash about her father.

"I'm sorry." Charlotte frowned, her fingers tapping on her thighs. "I didn't mean for you to feel like you had to take sides. It's not fair to you, and that wasn't my goal. I'll try not to do it again."

Adam nodded stiffly. "Thanks."

"Sure." Charlotte paused. "Dad told me about your mom. The whole story. I'm really, really sorry, Adam. I just wanted you to know that."

Adam's shoulders drooped—his body rigid. Motionless.

146

Charlotte crept from the stairs and stepped down onto the sidewalk. "Please, I'm on your side. We don't have to be best friends, but we've got to at least start working together. Let's not try to solve every problem in one night, but maybe dealing with this *together* will help. I'm going to take a walk. Want to come? It always makes me feel better."

Adam looked out at the lake and back at Charlotte. He frowned.

"Ditto." Jerking his head, he stepped from the porch. Rather than heading toward the waterfront path, though, he strode around the corner and south on Pine. Charlotte hurried to keep up. Adam thrust his hands in his pockets, and the bill of his baseball cap pushed into the wind. It reminded her of her first walk with Jake. She'd been just as prickly. In their similar pain, perhaps she and her half-brother weren't so different, after all.

"So, let's do the 'get to know you' thing," Charlotte said, wishing she'd grabbed a warmer jacket. He wouldn't wait if she asked to go back and get one.

"Whatever," Adam said.

Charlotte glanced at the mostly deserted cottages they passed along the way, noting only two houses showing signs of life—cars or interior lights—along their path.

"Maybe tell me about school?"

Adam shrugged. "What's to tell?"

"Do you like it? Do you like your teachers?"

"It's fine," Adam said, shrugging again. "They're fine."

Charlotte allowed the silence to envelop them once more, somewhat humored by his stoicism. He wasn't ready to talk. What teenager was?

They passed a paint-chipped white home with purple trim. It made up for its small stature with the wrap-around porches adorning more than half of the exterior, and at least a dozen bikes littered the front, even during the off-season.

"Clown cottage," Charlotte mumbled.

"What?"

"Clown cottage. When I was a kid, I always called that place the clown cottage, because of how many people go into it. Like a clown car, you know?"

"I get it," Adam said.

"So many people, and I could never figure out where they all slept. I'd see them on the screened porch sometimes, at night, but—"

"Nah," Adam said. "I think it's like that book by C.S. Lewis."

"Chronicles of Narnia?"

"Yep. They go in, but hardly anyone comes out, so I'm pretty sure they just disappear into a wardrobe and open a door to a different realm or something."

Charlotte laughed. "I like your backstory far better than mine. Very creative."

The siblings took a left and eventually wrapped back around to the waterfront, bottoming out at the west edge of the Hotel Lakeside.

"My parents were married here," Charlotte said. "It was a rainy day in May. Supposed to happen around the fountain, I guess, but they had to do it inside. Mom says she came down the staircase. I'd never do that. I'm so klutzy, I'd end up at the bottom of the steps in a pile of tulle. Two broken arms. Two broken legs. One broken head."

"Yeah? Well, my parents never married. So, there's that."

Silence.

"Crap. I'm so sorry, Adam. That's not what I meant—"

"I get it. You were trying to be funny." Adam picked up a rock from beside the path and let it fly over the water, skipping three times before sinking. "Dude, the broken arms and legs thing... that was decent."

Could this get any more awkward?

"Sorry. I don't know how much Dad has told you about me, but I'm not good at this." Charlotte waved her hand between them. "Socially, I basically suck. I'm not Chuck. Have never been Chuck.

148

Will never, ever, ever *be* Chuck. So, anything I say will probably be exactly what you don't want to hear. I'm terrible at this."

The look on Adam's face was disbelief.

"I only communicate well in writing. It's not intentional, *dude*. Just keeping it real."

"Wow." Adam smiled slightly. He shook his head and looked out at the water. "You're not kidding, are you?"

"I rarely kid. Sarcasm is more my thing."

"Yeah, me too."

Charlotte pulled her hands from her pockets and blew into them. There was a chill in the air—colder than normal for early November. She'd need to shop for warmer clothes if she really planned to stick it out until Thanksgiving.

"What sports do you play?" Charlotte said. "Baseball? Basketball? What's your go-to?"

"I'm better at baseball than anything else, so that's my favorite. I play basketball, too, and some pick-up soccer."

"I sucked at every sport I tried," Charlotte said. "The worst was cheer camp. When I was little, I'd play dress-up in Mom's old Biting Walleyes uniform. In sixth grade, I finally got to try out. It was a complete bust. I towered over everyone. Most of the girls had taken gymnastics or dance classes, but not me. I was so uncoordinated, I literally tripped over an imaginary line." Charlotte groaned. "It was bad. Really bad. Looks like you must have gotten the only athletic Sutton gene."

They paused at a bench along the waterfront, and Charlotte sat down. Adam joined her.

"So, do you want to be a professional athlete like Dad? I mean, I assume you do," Charlotte said. "If you're remotely as good as he was."

"I'm not." Adam shook his head. "And I don't. I'm not interested."

He sounded certain.

"Huh. Any idea what you *do* want to do after high school?" Charlotte said.

"Yeah." Adam tapped the journal he still held in his hand. "I'm pretty sure I'd like to write, just like you."

"Like Chuck," Charlotte murmured.

Adam looked down at his sneakers. "Yeah. I want to be a writer like you and Dad."

20

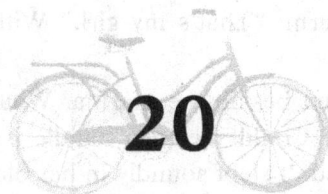

The days blurred, turning into a week and more. Charlotte adjusted to her father's schedule, continued her remote advertising work, and tiptoed around her sibling. She started to get the hang of things. Or thought she had.

Until Franco Bellimer stopped her in the parking lot of the marina on a Monday morning.

"We've got a problem, Charlotte. Your dad got a call from the printer. This week's issue was missing files, and Kate is handling it, but we need to cover the Bay Area School Board meeting tonight. Could you do it? I'm headed to two interviews later, and I just don't think Chuck is up to it. He's having a bad day."

Charlotte glanced at the door leading to *The Lakeside Line*. "Um, sure."

Bad day? What does that even mean?

"Pull the agenda off the website," Franco said. "They hold their meetings in the auditorium. We just need about 500 words on what's happening in the district this month. If there's anything about the budget or sports, that should work."

"I don't know, Mr. B. I haven't done any newswriting for years. Not since I was editor for the student newspaper in college."

Franco Bellimer arched a brow. "You're not nervous, are you? You'll be fine."

"Of course, I'll be fine. It's just—"

"What?"

Charlotte sighed. "Nothing. I'll do it."

He nudged her arm. "That's my girl." With a wave, Bellimer went to his car.

Charlotte hesitated beside the marina. What to expect behind Door Number Two? Could she even handle it when she was this tired? So far, she hadn't slept soundly in her old bed, often staring out the window well into the night—her brain unable to turn off until the wee hours. Like muck from the bottom of the lake during a storm, so many memories had stirred to the surface since she'd returned. She couldn't shrug off the weight of her father's health, and the relationship with her brother was confusing and complex.

She wanted a damned do-over or at least a moment to breathe.

Charlotte entered the hall and reached the entrance to the office. Suddenly, the door to The Surly Sturgeon slammed behind her.

"Morning, Charlie."

She turned and placed a hand on her hip.

"Charlotte." Jake grinned. "Sorry. I'll try harder." His hair stuck out in all directions, a disconnect from his neatly trimmed beard. Sydney trotted along beside him and immediately swerved to Charlotte for a pet.

She sunk her fingers into the animal's fur. "It's fine."

"I'll get it eventually," Jake said. "I promise."

The use of the nickname still annoyed Charlotte but, perhaps, not quite as much. Jake's smile dulled the edges. It was, quite simply, a very nice smile.

"Franco said that you're staying for a couple more weeks?"

Charlotte scratched Sydney behind an ear. "Yep. The agency is pretty cool about me working remotely, but I'm leaving as soon as I get things under control."

"Oh."

"Do you have a charter this morning?"

"Already done," Jake said. "It was at seven. I don't have anything else until after lunch. Thought I'd come see how you and your dad are getting along."

"Swimmingly."

Jake laughed. "She says with a pained expression. By the way, how was the doctor's appointment last week? I never got to ask."

"It could have gone better." Charlotte leaned a shoulder against the wall and told him what transpired during and after the appointment.

"Wow. You lost him? That's crazy."

Charlotte nodded. "Freaked me out. The neurologist wants to discuss medications, and I've got to talk with Dad about putting Mr. B in charge of the office."

Jake's face fell. "I'm so sorry. Sounds like the appointment *definitely* could have gone better."

"Yeah, and today is apparently a bad day."

"Hmmm. Chuck's bad days can be *very* bad. Let me help; we can handle him together."

"I'd appreciate that."

"I'm all yours."

Nodding, Charlotte opened the door to the office. To her surprise, Kate Fallow sat in the second office. Hammering away at her keyboard, Charlotte's previous high school classmate didn't take her eyes from her monitor. She fluttered her fingers in the air by way of greeting.

"Welcome back," Kate said. "Give me just a sec. I've gotta get this file to Printing Pro."

Chuck leaned back in his office chair, his feet planted on the floor and arms folded on his chest. He was staring out the window.

"Hey." Charlotte walked into his sightline. "How's it going?"

"What?" Her father looked up. He glanced beyond Charlotte. "You seen Franco?"

"He just left," Jake said.

"Mr. B went to an interview." Charlotte stuffed her gloves in a pocket and dropped her coat onto the hook behind the door. "How are things?"

"How are things?" Chuck scowled. "How are things? Jesus. Would be a hell of a lot better if people would stop asking me that. Why's everyone keep asking so many questions?"

"Sorry."

"Son of a bitch." Chuck's voice rose. "I'm tired of questions." He shook his head, leaned over, and rested his arms on his knees.

"Sorry, Chuck." Charlotte's stomach clenched. Their relationship had improved somewhat since her arrival. Yet, she'd so easily slipped back into calling him "Chuck"—the more natural fit than "Dad" ever would be.

Two steps forward. One step back.

It was exhausting.

Kate popped her head out her doorway. "We're good to go, Mr. Sutton. I sent the files to the printer. He'll be able to get it done so we can mail on time. Is that all you need from me today?"

Chuck nodded. "Yes."

He looked as tired as Charlotte felt.

"It's my fault," Chuck muttered. "I'm sorry I sent him the wrong files." He shoved his fingers through his hair, ruffling the black mess and making the coarse streaks of silver around his temples stand at attention. "I sent him the wrong damned files. The wrong files!" Throwing himself back in his chair, Chuck scratched the stubble on his chin—the rasp of sandpaper sending a chill crawling up Charlotte's neck. His anger was something foreign to her. He had rarely, if ever, raised his voice to anyone.

Chuck returned to looking out the window.

"It's all good, Mr. Sutton," Kate said. "Really. How about if I send the files from now on, since I do the layout? Would that help eliminate a step?"

Chuck nodded. "Thank you, Charlie. Perhaps it would."

Charlotte and Kate's eyes locked. He'd confused them.

Chuck swiveled in his chair, noticed Kate, and looked back at Charlotte. His gaze shifted again toward the window. "I'm sorry I caused you so much trouble."

"No worries, Mr. Sutton," Kate said. "Happy to help."

"I need more of that than you can give." Chuck closed his eyes. "A lot more."

Behind Chuck's back, Kate played a two-second game of charades, communicating that she needed to speak with Charlotte alone. Charlotte nodded.

She'd never seen her father like this. It wasn't just the anger and confusion. While she was growing up, even during the divorce, he'd always been so annoyingly positive. Hence the name Good-time Charlie.

But not today. Today, he seems defeated.

Charlotte gave Jake a look over her father's head.

"What can I do?" he said.

Charlotte turned Chuck's desktop computer around so it could be accessed from the opposite side. "You mind looking up the Bay Area School Board agenda for tonight's meeting while I talk with Kate for a few minutes? We haven't seen each other since graduation. Just want to catch up."

"No problem. I'll print it out for you." Jake fell into a chair and began typing away.

Charlotte stepped into Kate's office, closing the door behind her, and was immediately grabbed up in a hug.

Kate pulled back to appraise her with a crooked grin. "Hello, city girl."

"Hello, lake girl."

Only a couple of years younger than Charlotte, the buxom woman with a messy bun of straw-like hair appeared older. She wore faded blue jeans and a paint-splattered sweatshirt that displayed an anchor with the words "Let's get NAUTI."

"I'm so sorry about your dad," Kate said. "Today's been... rough."

"Does he get like this very often?"

"Sometimes."

Charlotte frowned. "That can't be easy."

"It's not so bad. Mr. B is a big help."

"I can't believe you're both working here," Charlotte said. "Almost like journalism class."

"I know, right? But these past few months haven't been nearly as fun."

"No, I guess not."

Kate returned to her desk chair. She tipped it back and plunked a sneaker on the corner of her desk and threw one ankle over the other.

"So, your dad had a doc appointment last week, yeah?"

"Yes." Charlotte slumped into the spare chair across from Kate and caught her up. "This is going to get worse. Much worse. I almost lost him, Kate. I found him having a beer by himself at Quarters. He didn't even know who I was."

"I'm so sorry."

"How's he been at the office?" Charlotte grimaced. "I mean, obviously, today isn't great."

"Most days, he just gets confused. He uses his notes. It's rare, but sometimes he gets angry, like today. It comes on really sudden. And your dad hasn't been bringing in any new advertisers. Word's getting around he's not well, and there've been complaints from the regulars. Chuck just hasn't been on his game."

"Crap." Charlotte gazed out the window. "What if you did ad

156

sales? You'd get commission, of course. Chuck can work something out. He's got the money."

Kate made a face. "Sales is *not* my thing." She motioned to her paint-splattered work attire. "Your dad is lucky I didn't show up in my pajamas today. I'd rather be behind the computer. I'm a keyboard nerd, not a salesman."

"Yeah." Charlotte did the math in her head. "I'll make some calls to the local shops. Maybe I can boost the ads myself in the next few weeks. What if you handled the administrative stuff, like the accounting? Dad shouldn't be doing it anymore."

"That'd work," Kate said. "I already deal with the advertisers' artwork, so adding billing wouldn't be hard. Why not? How many more hours you thinking? I'll take whatever you can give me. My partner and I are trying to save up for a house before we get married."

"Cool. Congratulations. Anyone I know?"

"Nah. Rachel is from Cleveland. She's a pilot I met at a diversity conference. We're trying to find a place to buy midway between here and the airport."

Charlotte nodded. "I'm not sure about hours. I'll look at the books and get back to you. We probably need someone full-time here at the office, to be honest. I didn't plan on staying much past Thanksgiving. I bought myself some extra time. The agency I'm with has me doing remote work, but I've got to get back as soon as possible. It's just a lot."

"We'll do whatever needs done," Kate said. "You know that, right? Jake and Franco and Bea and I—we'll help you get through this."

Tears welled beneath Charlotte's lids. She couldn't imagine asking for the same help from her Pittsburgh city neighbors.

"Thanks. I really appreciate the support. Look, I know we haven't talked in years, but it's really great to see you again."

Kate smiled. "You too. What the heck took you so long to come back for a visit?"

"Too many reasons to explain."

"Well, I'm glad you're here." Kate shut down her computer and grabbed her coat. She pulled out her phone. "I'll give you my number in case you need me for anything. We should go for drinks or something. Lots to catch up on."

Charlotte added Kate to her contacts. "Sounds great."

"Well, I gotta get going." Kate threw her laptop into a bag. "My parents are expecting me to help finish painting their spare bedroom this afternoon."

Charlotte followed Kate into the main office. Chuck was still peering out the window.

"See ya'." Kate let herself out.

Jake motioned for Charlotte. "Here's the agenda. Doesn't look like anything too crazy. They're talking about the plans for the high school renovation. Some people might ask questions about that."

"Okay," Charlotte said. "Do the locals want it?"

"Not if it will cost too much," Chuck mumbled.

Charlotte lightly tapped her father's shoulder. "Dad, you cover the school board meetings every month, right?"

It took a moment for Chuck to focus. "Yes."

"Has the Bay Area renovation been a big deal?"

"Yes." Chuck slowly turned in his chair to face them. "The capital improvement budget might... raise some questions." He paused, his words coming with effort, like he had to re-order them in his brain. "Bay Area has tourist money coming in, but we... the paper has to tell the locals what it will cost, down the road."

"Franco wants me to cover today's meeting." Charlotte exchanged a look with Jake. "Since you're tired."

"Yeah, I am tired." Chuck turned again toward the window. "But we'll go together. You drive, Charlie. I'll introduce you around. That way no one will think it's odd you are covering the meetings from now on."

I'm not going to be here that long. I can't.

"Sure, Dad."

Jake looked at his phone and stood. "Sorry, but I've got to go. I need to get ready for my next charter. Do you want something for lunch, Chuck? Bea made homemade perogies for the daily special. I think she put cabbage and bacon in 'em."

"No thanks, kid."

"You've got this," Jake said, turning toward Charlotte. His eyes, sea blue with flecks of copper, reminded Charlotte of her father's Sunfish, Old Betty, the sailboat she'd spent hours on as a child.

"Thanks."

"Oh, and how about dinner tonight at the bar after your meeting?"

A bead of sweat broke out on Charlotte's forehead. Was it a date? A date with Jake sounded far more appealing than a date with Jim Stanner, despite the new six-pack abs.

"Um, sure."

"Great."

"See you then." Jake sidled out the door.

Chuck leaned back in his chair, his gaze lost to the deserted marina parking lot. His chin drifted toward his chest.

"Let me know when the proofs come back from the printer, Kate."

21

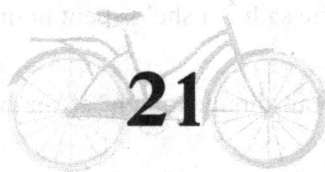

Chuck's anger abated, and he remained quiet the rest of the day. He eventually fell asleep in his chair for an afternoon nap.

Charlotte dived into her father's computer, trying to make sense of the unorganized files and eventually finding two different working folders—similarly named—for the next week's issue. With a paper at the printer and another deadline looming, she took a crack at editing the content.

As a child, she'd always liked reading her father's writing, even when she didn't really understand sports. Ten years had not changed that, though she found many misspellings and incomplete sentences, further proof the Alzheimer's had started to impact Chuck's work. Charlotte also turned to edit Franco's feature about ice-fishing, a winter activity she remembered enjoying with her father when she was quite young. The memory made her smile.

With her father a silent presence throughout the process, Charlotte plugged away for more than three hours, doing the work of editor of a small-town newspaper.

She hadn't wanted or expected to enjoy the process.

Nor had she expected to feel like she belonged, for the first time ever, in Lakeside, Ohio.

*   *   *   *   *

Later that day, she pulled into a parking space at Bay Area High School. With its Biting Walleyes logo and metal walleye sculpture in the entry, the building looked like it had changed not at all since Charlotte's departure.

The predictability annoyed her and gave her a warm, fuzzy feeling. Mostly the first. A bit of the latter.

"We're here." Charlotte killed the engine and nudged her father's elbow. "You ready?"

"Almost." Chuck placed his briefcase on his lap. He reached inside, pulled a small voice recorder from a pocket, and handed the device to his daughter. "Nine school board directors, the superintendent, the board attorney, and various administrative staff will attend. They sit at a long table. Until you get to know them, the easiest way to remember who's talking is to take a picture with your phone, number them left to right, and jot down the person's number in your notes." Chuck nodded, all business. "If you note the speaker number and time on the recorder, you'll be able to find the complete quote later and know who's talking."

Charlotte shook her head. "Wow. Okay. Wouldn't it be just as easy to use the recorder on my phone?"

"Whatever you're comfortable with. Personally, I still like the old-school recorder."

"That might be because you are—"

"Old? Yeah, maybe, kid."

Charlotte laughed. Her father had woken from his nap refreshed and focused. There was a buzzing energy about him now, like he was gearing up for an interview with a famous athlete instead of covering the local school district's typical monthly business.

"I've been doing this a long time," Chuck said. "Whether your old man's losing his marbles or not, some things take a long time to forget." He patted Charlotte's knee. "Let's go break in my new star reporter."

161

Swept up in the moment, Charlotte let her father lead the way. The warmth of his encouragement filled her, though his opinion had always mattered so much more than it should. Why did she care? It was weird to hear his praise, now, after so many years. Weirder, still, to trail behind him as if they were a writing team.

Charlotte hung back, allowing Chuck to enter the auditorium first. The space had received a makeover since her graduation—new seats and a blue, velveteen curtain. People dotted the auditorium chairs closest to the stage, where three long tables arched in a wide "U" with the open side facing the audience. At each chair had been placed a placard with a name and a microphone.

Chuck strode down the left aisle and dropped into a chair at a separate table reserved for reporters. Charlotte followed.

She could hear the sounds of people entering and filling in behind her, but no one else joined them at the media table and she did not turn around. Woefully exposed, sitting next to her father, she did not want anyone to recognize her, just yet. Staying away for a decade was as good a reason as any for the locals to be curious, but she needed time to gird herself for the questions she might receive. And there *would* be questions.

Board members began mounting the auditorium stairs. A man in a work shirt and cargo pants strode across the stage, tapped each microphone, and descended to a podium on the audience level. Flicking a switch, he tested the podium microphone. With a yank of his britches, he proceeded up their aisle. Charlotte caught a whiff of cigarettes and fried food as he passed.

She leaned in to her father. "What does a girl have to do to get paid in Netty's chili dogs around here? I've got a craving."

Chuck's snort startled the woman sitting across the aisle.

He patted Charlotte's knee. "If you are a good daughter, I will take you for dinner sometime this spring, after they open back up for season."

"That would be great."

Or it would be if she were going to be around to take him up on his offer. Charlotte did not have the heart to break it to him; the day had been rough enough.

"You're going to dinner with Jake later, right? If it were me, I'd order the wings, double-fried and extra crispy with garlic parm sauce on the side, but I suppose that's not a great suggestion for a first date."

Charlotte smiled. He remembered. Even bad days could have good moments.

"It's not a date. Thanks, though. I had almost forgotten."

"Remember what you can," Chuck said, tapping Charlotte's hand. "Forgetting is a right pisser, kid. And, for the record, Jake's a good boy—husband material."

"For real? What are you, my matchmaker?"

"Just looking out for my little girl. Best turn on the recorder now, Charlie. The superintendent will give her report just after they do the Pledge of Allegiance."

"How long will this take?"

"All depends on if anyone has something to bitch about. With Monday night football, I'd expect to be out of here in less than an hour."

Charlotte pulled out her notebook and set the recorder on the table.

Superintendent Dr. Openheimer, a robust woman with glasses, prominent teeth, and pale hair swept into a bun, had little to say in her report to the board members. Of small note, she thanked the Walleyes Friends Association for providing a grant for repairs to the side parking lot.

Glancing at the recorder to confirm it was on, Charlotte listened to the financial report, given by a director who spent several minutes spewing numbers and referencing a spreadsheet. He talked way too fast for Charlotte to keep up with her notes. The board had provided an info packet on the district website, though, along with the agenda

163

and back-up materials. More concerning was the real possibility she'd fall asleep writing a story on the dry content.

After the financial report, Charlotte suffered through the human resources report, the facilities report, the technology report, the special education report, and, surprisingly, a very short explanation of the proposed renovation budget. One of the final agenda items included an effusive "thanks for hiring me" speech by the high school principal—a squat Mr. Hallicott with the baby-faced appearance of someone yet to get his driver's license. Times had changed. He was nothing like Charlotte's previous high school principal, a man in his eighties who waited 20 years too long to retire.

"Story on the new principal?" Charlotte whispered in Chuck's ear.

"That's right, kid. And talk to Kate about getting a proper picture."

Following Mr. Hallicott, audience members wishing to address the board were asked to step forward. A shuffling of seats and click-clack of footsteps filtered forward from behind Charlotte.

Dana, dressed in black pants and a turtleneck, walked down the aisle. A little blond girl wearing a tutu and a fuzzy pink sweater held her hand and skipped along beside her. Dana approached the podium and tapped the microphone. It popped static, and she took a step back.

"State your name and address for the record, please," the board secretary said.

"Dana Fletcher McKenzie. This is my daughter, Trinity. We live at 617 Opal Drive, Lakeside Marblehead."

"Thank you, Mrs. McKenzie. You may proceed."

Dana pulled a piece of paper from her bag. "Sorry. I'm a little nervous, so I'll just read this." She smoothed the creases and cleared her throat. "My husband, Mike McKenzie, a graduate of Bay Area High School, lost his life protecting a children's center overseas two years ago. The suicide bomber took out a city block, killing my husband and more than half of his squad, plus almost 30 children and teachers. We live in different times. For the safety of our students, I request that the board consider additional security measures and threat training at each of the district's school buildings."

Charlotte straightened, her pencil flying across her notebook.

"Across the state and nationwide, schools are seeing a rise in violence," Dana said. "School and public shootings, bomb scares, and so on, are no longer something that just happens in the big cities or across international borders. Research indicates more than half the incidents of school violence in the U.S., this past year, occurred in less than a dozen states. Ohio and our neighbor, Pennsylvania, have fallen within that statistic in the past decade. For the sake of our children, I feel a review of our safety protocols and additional threat training and education is in the best interest of my daughter Trinity and the other children of this community." Dana let out a breath. "Thank you."

"Are there any questions for Mrs. McKenzie?" the board secretary asked.

"Not at this time," Superintendent Openheimer said. "Thank you for your suggestions. We will take them under advisement and discuss them during our executive session."

Dana nodded. Trinity, with a smile wide enough to light up The Surly Sturgeon, preceded her up the aisle. As they passed, Dana grinned, gave Charlotte two thumbs up, and kept walking.

"Wow," Charlotte said. "That was simply fantastic."

"She did quite well," Chuck said. "Pay attention. This could get interesting."

Additional members of the community approached the microphone. A neighbor of the high school discussed the noise level of the football games, and the father of a middle school band member requested new tubas. Finally, an older fellow made his way down the aisle. He carried a hat in a gnarled hand and clutched a cane with his other. Charlotte put him at 90, give or take a decade.

"Ronald Brewster, 6464 Beach Road, Lakeside Marblehead."

"Thank you, Mr. Brewster. Proceed."

165

Mr. Brewster cleared his throat.

"Do you need a drink of water, Mr. Brewster?" the board secretary said.

"Thank you, no," Brewster said. "I first wish to offer Mrs. McKenzie my condolences for the loss of her husband and to thank him, posthumously, for his service to our country. However, as much as Mrs. McKenzie's idea is admirable, in theory and intent, I must most adamantly object to the added expense the community would incur with this threat training nonsense. Our taxes are high enough as it is. We live in a small community—a safe community. Truth be told, I haven't locked my doors in more than 70 years. Why fix what ain't broke, I always say. No offense to Mrs. McKenzie."

A buzz of dissent and murmurs filtered behind Charlotte.

"Thank you for your input, Mr. Brewster," Superintendent Openheimer said. "We will take your suggestions under advisement and discuss them during our executive session."

"Thank you kindly." The man hobbled to a seat on the opposite aisle and slumped down in disgust. The meeting ended shortly thereafter.

"That was more interesting than I expected," Charlotte said.

"Yeah, well, that's the local news," Chuck said, patting her hand. "Now go ask questions."

"Gotcha."

Charlotte approached the principal. "Hi. I'm Charlotte Sutton. I'm a Bay Area grad, and my dad, Editor Chuck Sutton, would like me to do a feature on you for *The Lakeside Line*. Is there a time we could meet?"

Mr. Hallicott took a very quick scan of Charlotte, ending with him looking up her nose. "Sure, Miss Sutton." He bent to his phone. "Tomorrow? Eleven o'clock?"

Charlotte nodded, making a note of the appointment. "I'll see you then. Our photographer, Kate Fallow, will call you, or a professional headshot would work fine, too."

Mr. Hallicott smiled. "Great. I look forward to our chat."

"Same."

"Well, if it isn't Charlie Sutton," chortled a high, sing-songy voice.

"Oh, Lord," Charlotte muttered. "If you'll excuse me, Mr. Hallicott?" The principal nodded, and Charlotte turned to witness Tipsy Levine careen down the aisle. The retired secretary still wore a sheer blouse and stiletto heels, a decade later. She had swapped her short skirts for skinny jeans.

"Carnegie Mellon graduate. Published writer. My, my. Well done, child. The apple doesn't fall far from the tree." Tipsy's red pump took a turn, and, with cat-like reflexes, Chuck threw out an arm and caught her. Tipsy didn't mind a bit. She leaned, seconds too long, against Chuck, her wrinkled bosoms squished and heaving between the two of them like the downy heads of Siamese twins. "Oh, thank you, Chuck. Whoopsie."

Chuck grinned. "The pleasure was mine, Ellie."

Charlotte sighed. "Hi, Ms. Levine."

"Job shadowing your dad, hmmm?" Tipsy reached a manicured hand out and trailed it down Chuck's sleeve. "We can *all* learn a lot from him, I bet."

"Sure."

"We're so blessed to have a famous author in our midst. Sooo blessed."

Chuck squeezed the woman's hand. "You're too kind, Ellie."

This. This is why I left.

"Nice to see you, Ms. Levine." Charlotte turned. "You haven't changed a bit."

22

HIGH SCHOOL

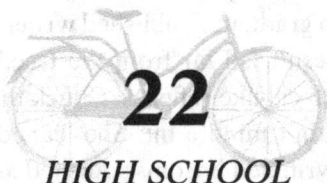

Charlotte sat in the next-to-last line of Bay Area High School graduates. A few around her sniffled into tissues. Not Charlotte, of course. What was there to cry about?

"Amelia Angelina Evans."

"Joel David Flynn."

Each student in Bay Area blue made his or her way onto the stage, walked across to the podium, shook hands with the superintendent, and accepted a diploma. Many waved and carried on to parents and friends in the auditorium.

"Bri Elizabeth Heiney."

An unfortunate name for Bri, no fat-bottom-girl.

"Dana Elianna Fletcher."

Clapping and whistles erupted from the audience.

Charlotte rolled her eyes. The senior popularity contest was scored strictly by the loudness of each graduate's fan club. Dana would get at least a bronze medal. Of course, she'd probably get knocked down a notch or two on the podium by Class President Justin Jespers III. Justin publicly despised people who forgot the III, distinguishing him from his dad, Justin Jespers, Jr., an accountant who had ended up in prison for tax evasion.

The III had much higher aspirations. Gold medal, for sure.

"They deserve a standing 'O,' Char," Sammy whispered over his shoulder. "It's a miracle they graduated at all."

"Truth," Charlotte said.

"Shhh," Ms. Levine hissed from the end of Charlotte's row. "No talking."

The middle school secretary had gotten a promotion to the high school just in time to usher Charlotte into adulthood. That Tipsy had never been fired for unprofessional attire and equally unprofessional student "counseling" was a sad state of educational affairs, in Charlotte's humble opinion.

"We're up, Macon," the boy next to Sammy said. The line of students in front of Charlotte stood.

"Love," Charlotte said, earning another glare from Ms. Levine. "See ya' on the other side."

Sammy, still the shortest guy in their class of only 137, stood in front of the tallest classmate to matriculate, star quarterback Mike McKenzie. Heat crept to Charlotte's cheeks and she dismissed the ridiculous idea that she could, or ever would, be with someone like Mike. He was out of her league and firmly in Dana's pocket.

After receiving his diploma, Sammy did not do a touchdown dance or raise the roof or any of the previous students' celebratory nonsense. He gave a nod to the crowd and accepted the mild clapping reserved for the new kid in town. Five years a Biting Walleye was still considered practically a summer tourist. Moments later, Tipsy Levine leaned over the football player at the end of Charlotte's row.

"Rise."

Charlotte followed Amber Sundry, the class goth with more piercings than there were high school faculty.

Tara "Pops" Thomas, a girl with a bubblegum fetish, nudged Charlotte from behind. "Hurry up, Tree."

"Ricky Jonathon Reidenbacher."

Stupid nicknames. Nicki "The Hickey" had outed Ricky as "The Quickie" in their sophomore year. How embarrassing.

Charlotte grinned a little too wide as she approached the aisle. Ms. Levine frowned and ushered her into the graduation line. Most students scratched or shuffled. They twisted to look for their parents and whispered to their neighbors. Charlotte knew where her mother and Sammy's mother were sitting. Barely paying any attention to the classmates graduating ahead of her, Charlotte kept her eye on Amber's black asymmetrical bob, shaved on the left side. If Charlotte closed one eye then the other, she could almost convince herself Amber was actually two different people.

Two different strangers.

That's the way she thought of her peers. None had taken the time to see her as anything but The Tree. The realization that she had not gotten to know them either flitted into, and just as quickly out of, Charlotte's head. A fly to be swatted away.

Who cares?

Charlotte mounted the stairs.

"Charlotte Anne Sutton."

The superintendent's palm was moist and warm. Charlotte accepted her diploma and looked out, seeking familiar faces in the crowd.

There. Mama Macon and Mom.

And Chuck.

Charlotte sucked in a breath. Her father had made it and surprised her. He'd said he'd be traveling and wouldn't be home. Charlotte's heart beat faster. A smile jumped to her lips and fell away just as quickly as the hand she'd begun to raise in greeting.

Not Chuck.

The seat beside Elise Sutton was filled by another stranger—a gentleman who looked very much like her father.

But not Chuck.

Of course, not Chuck.

At least *some* kid's father had shown up.

"Whoop, whoop. Go, Char," Sammy yelled from the seats.

Charlotte ducked her head and continued down the steps and back to her chair. She leaned over and rapped Sammy's mortarboard with her diploma, as a "thank you" for the shout-out.

Turning the rolled paper over in her hands and pulling the blue ribbon off one end, she unfurled the proof of her accomplishment—a poorly-copied facsimile of the actual diploma, to be mailed to Charlotte a week or two later in a fancy, cardboard frame.

She stared at her name.

Charlotte Anne Sutton.

Charlotte thought about the stranger—some kid's father who had shown up in Chuck's place. She didn't feel weepy or sad or even particularly happy. She didn't *feel* anything.

None of it mattered.

Her parents were divorced. She had graduated. She would move on. There was absolutely nothing to keep her in this little town with its little people. She was The Tree, after all, just as they'd forced upon her.

It would be fine. She didn't feel weepy or sad. What she felt, more or less, was relieved.

There's got to be something bigger than this.

23

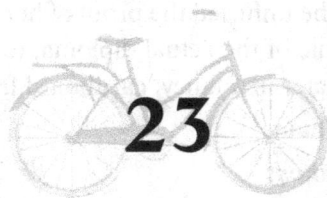

Sorry Sorry Sorry Sorry Sorry Sorry—

Charlotte pressed send. Sammy could ignore her texts only so long. How many sorries would it take?

She pulled open the door to The Surly Sturgeon and scanned the room. Jake sat at the bar. The game was several minutes into its first quarter, and the place only hosted about a dozen patrons. Charlotte vaguely recognized three of them, in addition to Franco Bellimer, who perched at his favorite table watching Bea play darts with herself. He gave Charlotte a wave, which she returned. In the short time she'd been back in town, she'd been in the bar at least three or four times. Did that make her a regular?

Dismissing the ridiculous thought, she plopped into the seat next to Jake.

"Phew, getting crowded in here. Glad I beat the rush. How many Cleveland touchdowns did I miss?"

"What? They haven't—"

"Joking." Charlotte rolled her eyes.

Jake threw his arms up, referee style. "We've graduated to jokes."

"All right, settle down." Charlotte smiled. "Don't hurt yourself."

Dana bussed a table near the window. She had changed out of her conservative, talking-to-the-school-board clothes and into a team shirt with a plunging neckline. Stuffing a tip into her pocket, she swiped the surface with a rag. Two bottle-blonde women, about Charlotte's age, sipped wine at a high-top in the corner. They looked familiar; perhaps she'd seen them at the school board meeting. Eyeing Dana, both chattered away with quiet intensity. Whether they were dishing about Dana's tip-enhancing waitress get-up or her request for school security protocols, Charlotte couldn't guess. The red-wine drinker, a heavy woman with equally heavy makeup, met Charlotte's gaze and turned her chair, leaning in to her too-skinny, pasty-pale, white-wine-drinking buddy, who looked over her shoulder.

"What can I get you to drink?" Dana tossed a coaster on the counter.

"Whatever seasonal craft beer you have on tap," Charlotte said. "Porter? Or a stout?"

"Give the city girl that new frou-frou shit Porch Kitty Brewing just saddled us with," Bea said. She winged another dart in the corner, striking the board just south of a bullseye. "None of my regulars will drink frou-frou. Why I let them damn local startup brewers talk me into the fancy stuff, I'll never know." The Surly Sturgeon owner whipped another projectile. "Effing dart. Get in there, ya' worthless piece of shit."

"On it, boss." Dana grinned at Charlotte. "Don't mind Bea. She actually loves the local brewers. It's a really good beer. Want another, Jake?"

"Yes, please."

Dana ducked behind the bar and returned with a dark ale for Charlotte and a pale draft for Jake.

"That was some crazy meeting, huh?" Dana nodded at Charlotte. "I was so nervous. I was worried Mr. Brewster was going to give me a smack with his cane after, but he's so slow, I beat him out the door."

"He should be happy you care," Charlotte said. "In Pittsburgh, a student took a knife into a high school. Hurt a lot of people in less than 15 minutes. It was awful. I had to cover the kid's court case and interview the victims for my college newspaper. Fortunately, no one was killed, but the school security doubled after that. It's just typical now, I guess."

Dana frowned. "It shouldn't be. Not around here, anyway."

"No. It shouldn't. When I write the story, I'll have to give both sides," Charlotte said, "but I thought you did awesome."

"Thanks. That means a lot, coming from you."

"Your little girl is super cute. How old is she again?"

"Trinity just turned six. She's in kindergarten this year." Dana shook her head. "She's growing up so fast." She pulled napkins from her pocket, plopped them in front of Charlotte, and disappeared back into the kitchen.

People change, but Charlotte had not expected to find herself sympathizing with her enemy—a widow and single mother. She hadn't known Dana very well back in the day. Nor had Dana bothered to know her. Did the woman now deserve her friendship? Charlotte shook her head. Second chances were a hard thing to give.

"What's the story?" Jake said. "What did Dana have to say at the meeting?"

Charlotte explained.

"Wow. It takes guts to speak up."

"Yeah. Chuck thinks she has a 50/50 chance of getting what she wants."

"I would have hoped for better than that."

Charlotte shrugged. "The cost is the biggest issue."

"True." Jake tapped his glass. "Money is tight. Even Bea has raised her prices in the last year."

"Inflation, I guess." Charlotte took a sip. Her beer tasted faintly of fig, berry, and cinnamon. "Frou-frou or not, I like it, Bea."

Bea glanced over. "It's all yours, city girl. I can't give it away."

She released multiple darts in quick succession without facing the board. "For love of money and the devil's balls! Get in there, ya' worthless piece of shit."

"She's something." Jake leaned in, pressing his shoulder, solid and muscular, against Charlotte's own. A heat flowed straight down her mid-section. She shifted in her chair, feeling the absence of his arm even more acutely.

"For sure."

Charlotte grasped for something to say to fill the space she'd left between them.

Bea earned a bullseye, and Bellimer practically clapped himself silly.

"Oh, my gosh. I think Mr. B has a thing," Charlotte said, motioning.

"With Bea?" Jake nodded. "It's been going on for a while now, I think. He keeps asking her out, and she keeps saying 'no.' No idea why. I think they were made for each other."

"Could it be the age difference?" Charlotte said. "She's what? Maybe seven or eight years older than him?"

"Probably. Franco doesn't care, though, so why should she?"

"Fair." Charlotte turned in her chair.

Jake whispered in her ear, "They're both so stubborn, I don't think either of them will give in anytime soon. Minds are made up."

"That's too bad." Charlotte swallowed. His breath warmed her cheek.

"Yep," he said. "You can't catch what doesn't want to be caught."

"I suppose not."

"Well, unless you're a fisherman. Sometimes, a fisherman can outwit the enemy. Just got to be patient, is all."

"I guess I should be glad I'm not a fish," Charlotte said.

"Perhaps."

She briefly met Jake's gaze. He grinned.

"Soooo, next topic," Charlotte said. "Is the charter business your only job, or do you still work on the algae bloom problem?"

Jake pulled his phone from his pocket and quickly scanned through his photos.

"Here." He thrust a picture beneath Charlotte's nose. The almost fluorescent hue of a patch of algae, inches from two ducks and a row of ducklings, pooled across the surface of the water like an oil spill.

"I've been doing research, if you want to call it that, every time I go out on the boat. I took a lot of pictures this past summer, jotting down the coordinates of problem areas. Of course, everything moves with the wind, and some years we've thought the problem was solved. It's been kind of interesting. There's a new start-up organization working on this—Lake Erie Water Wellness Initiative. I'm hoping to get in on it. I submitted my resume last week, and if I'm lucky, funding will pay for someone like me. I mean, with the charter business, I'm on the lake. Why not take advantage of a biologist already in the field?"

Charlotte scrolled through Jake's pictures. "It's cool... what you're doing."

"I love Lake Erie."

"Me, too. It's what I missed most."

"Without the lake, this area would lose its livelihood. Businesses would shut down. People would go broke. This is our home, and everyone should take care of it."

Charlotte had sailed around the Lake Erie islands countless times. She'd spent entire days swimming off the Lakeside dock. On the water, or in it, she'd found peace. The lake had been one of the single most impactful aspects of her life.

"Maybe the newspaper should do an article."

"Chuck ran a story when Lakeside added an in-ground pool. With the algae, it was a smart move," Jake said. "A few of us science nerds spoke up in support of it."

"Maybe he should do a piece on the impact to businesses," Charlotte said. "Heck, I'd want to write that, if Chuck doesn't."

"I thought you weren't going to stick around." Jake nudged her shoulder.

Charlotte nudged back. "I'm not."

"That's a shame. You're going to miss out on Bea throwing her effing darts."

"Yes, there's that." Charlotte's gaze sought Jake's. He had kind eyes. Gentle. She liked them very much.

"So, enough about my tree-hugger ways. Tell me why you didn't come home for 10 years. Was it just because you and Chuck don't get along?"

So much for keeping it light.

Charlotte weighed her words. "Honestly, other than the lake, there was nothing left for me here." Her voice dropped. "Nothing, really, to come back to. No one cared I was gone—certainly not my father."

"Why would you think that? Your dad is thrilled you're back. *Every* person I know is. Franco, Dana, Kate, Bea, everyone."

"Bea? Are you sure? Because I'm pretty certain she can't stand me."

"Bea can't stand *anyone.*" Jake shrugged. "But she gives you crap about frou-frou beer. She obviously likes you."

"So, I should be honored?" Charlotte raised her beer for a celebratory toast and tipped it back, letting the cool brew wash down her throat. Feeling Jake's stare, she plunked the still-half-full drink back on the bar. She toyed with her silverware rolled in a napkin and spun the bundle like a bottle at a middle school party. It petered to a stop, pointing between two of the oldsters across from her. One shoved his work sleeves above his elbows, his calloused hands and nails dark from a day of physical labor at the nearby quarry. The other, a businessman, tapped his earphone speaker and stared into his beer. Was he listening to a call or contemplating something drastic?

She didn't care. She had no intention of sticking around to find out, as Jake suggested.

The less I know about these people, the better.

Dana returned to take their orders. Charlotte opted for the perch sandwich, Jake the shrimp basket. With a nod, she left them alone again.

"Do you think the reasons you chose to stay away still apply?" Jake said. "I mean, everybody changes. It's been a decade. Lakeside probably hasn't changed much in that time, but the people have. I bet you have, and I bet your dad has, too."

Charlotte's chest tightened with the reminder of her father and the unwelcome responsibility with which she'd been saddled. Why must she justify her choices? She shouldn't have to.

"I left because I didn't have a very easy time here."

Jake took a sip and waited.

"I never fit in, and Chuck wasn't around much. He was a sports writer before he wrote *Smokin' Smokey Joe*, and his job took him all over." Charlotte shrugged. "He did features for sports magazines and for all the major channels. When the book came out, he was gone even more to promote it. Writing was the thing I thought was coolest about my dad. It was also the thing that kept him away so much, and that was really hard for me."

Jake nodded. "I get that."

"But when he *was* around, it was all about sports. He and Adam might have that in common, but I was a disappointment to Chuck. I hated it. All I really wanted to do was write."

"Huh. Just like him."

"I suppose so." Charlotte took another sip of her beer.

"Well, it sure seems like you're good at it."

Charlotte spun the silverware again, watching the blur of white and silver rotate around and around. "Franco Bellimer told me I was the best student he'd ever had, but I can't ever remember my own father reading anything I wrote. He couldn't have cared less."

"You don't really believe that, do you?" Jake gently tapped Charlotte's forearm.

178

"What's not to believe? I graduated with a Bachelor of Arts degree in Creative Writing from Carnegie Mellon, summa cum laude. Chuck didn't even show up. He was never proud of the one thing I could do well. I've always thought it was because he didn't want anyone to take the attention away from himself."

"Nope," Jake shook his head. "I don't believe that. Chuck is so proud of you. He never shuts up about you. Every time you're published, your dad brags about it in his newspaper column and has Kate add the link to his website. You're not the only one who writes amazing essays. His stories about you and Adam, and being a proud parent who's never been very good at parenting, show how much he cares. Why do you think everyone is so happy to see you? We've been living your life with you. We know you through your writing and through his. You being back is like meeting a long-lost friend for the first time."

"Chuck writes essays about parenting? You've got to be kidding."

"I'm not. You can't tell me you haven't read them?"

"Of course not. I doubt my father has ever actually read anything I've written, either. I just found out my mom was sending him my stories, but—"

"I'm telling you. He's read them." Jake tapped his phone, and Chuck's website popped up. "Everyone has. See?"

"I don't understand. I didn't—"

Jake pointed. "He's posted all your links. Bottom right corner."

Charlotte gasped. When reviewing Chuck's website, she'd not opened the tab she assumed featured only his sports articles. Why would she want to read what had caused the divide between her and her father, in the first place?

She clicked, and a page entitled "Sutton's Choices" flooded the screen. Her father's headshot sat off to the left. A picture of Charlotte when she was very young, on the lake in a sailboat, graced the right side. Beneath them, centered, lay a shot of Adam in his baseball uniform. Charlotte clicked on Chuck's picture. It led to a link to purchase his book *"Smokin' Smokey Joe."* He'd also listed his essays—the most recent entitled "Living Alone Together." A quick skim of the contents revealed it was about raising a teenager without a mother.

Oh. My. God.

If Charlotte had followed her father's website, she'd have known she had a brother.

"It's all here. About Adam," Charlotte muttered. "How could he?"

As she scrolled further down, Charlotte discovered a story about her father teaching her to sail, a humor piece about throwing out the first pitch at the Cleveland stadium, a rendering of the Christmas morning Charlotte received her dollhouse, and multiple stories of her brother's sports exploits.

Charlotte backed out and clicked on her own picture, which led to a list of her own essay links. She clicked on the first one, and a story she had done for *The New Yorker* appeared on the screen.

That can't be right.

Her brain fuzzy, Charlotte clicked on another, and another. Her father had every link to every article she'd ever written, no matter how mundane.

"He's got all my stories."

"Yep. I've been trying to tell you."

You've read them, too?"

"*All* of them. Everyone has. Even the story about hating your hair and letting your friend cut it all off for the first time." Jake laughed, a deep, throaty, from-the-toes laugh. "Funny stuff, actually. I wasn't quite sure where that story was going. Thought maybe it was your first—"

"Oh, dear god. It was just supposed to be a funny set-up. I didn't think anyone I knew would ever read it."

Charlotte handed Jake his phone and laid her forehead down on her arms, pressing her nose into the bar napkin. It smelled faintly of stale fryer grease. Chuck's children were the feature story. And the whole damned town had been reading.

All of it. All of her.

"Did you think no one back home remembers you?" Jake tapped her lightly on the elbow. "You're practically a celebrity."

Charlotte fell back in her chair, placing both hands on her ears.

She couldn't unhear it, no matter how much she'd like to.

"What's wrong? You should be happy."

Dana came through the kitchen doors with two plates in her hands. "Here ya' go." She looked from one to the other. "Yeah, um, sorry to interrupt. Anyone need anything else?"

"Thanks, Dana." Jake grabbed the ketchup bottle. "I'm good."

"Another beer, please?" Charlotte said. "Gonna need it."

"No problem. I'll check on my other tables and grab you one." Smiling, Dana waved a hand in the air, encompassing them both. "In the meantime, I'll leave you to... this."

She departed, and they ate in silence. Charlotte kept rolling around the implications of what Jake had just shown her. If all of Lakeside and Marblehead Peninsula had been reading stories about her, written by her father, she couldn't have fared too badly. He'd want to look good to the public by making her childhood sound charming and whimsical. Her articles, however, were about growing up an insecure child in a split family with a famous father, a lack of athletic skill, and a burning desire to leave home.

Far from whimsical. Raw, even—particularly the ones about how she was bullied.

She'd never expected anyone she knew to ever read her stuff. In a few of her essays, she'd called people out by name, particularly those who had called her The Tree all through middle and high school. She'd also published a piece about her trip to the principal's office and the peer bully buddy system. She could only imagine what Dana and Tipsy Levine must think. How was Dana still speaking to her?

Maybe the article had illuminated how the cheerleader had treated others, back then—shamed her for being the bully she was? Maybe *that* was why she was being so nice now. Tipsy had not changed, though. Had Chuck ever taken the secretary up on her signals? She sure hoped not.

"Do you happen to know who the high school principal's secretary is, now that Ms. Levine retired?" Charlotte said.

Jake cocked his head. "No. Why?"

"No reason."

"Mmm, okay." Jake took another pull from his beer. "I won't pretend I understood that question."

"Probably best."

Silence filled the space between them. Not entirely awkward, but awkward enough.

"I'm complicated," she mumbled. "Best not to read too much into it."

"I see. Well, it's a good thing I don't mind complicated. Keeps me entertained." Jake gave her a side glance as he pulled the tab out of a tumbler on the bartender's ledge. "So, you're still going back to Pittsburgh, huh?"

Charlotte nodded. "That's the plan. I have a call scheduled with my boss tomorrow to talk about my next project. How much do I owe?"

"Nah, I got this." Jake's lips lifted into a half smile, and he threw some bills down. "I invited you."

"Thanks."

Date. Definitely a date. Dad was right.

"Want to walk on the dock before heading in?"

Charlotte's stomach fluttered. "Sure."

"You're pretty amenable tonight. I'm glad you've stopped running away with only your rocker for company."

"Technically, the rocker isn't mine. I was stealing it." Charlotte smiled. "That's a pretty lofty vocabulary word, by the way. Amenable. I like it."

"I do have a college degree, you know."

"Oh, of course. That's not what I meant. Please, don't—"

Jake shoved his shoulder against Charlotte's again, sending another ripple of heat down her body. "Relax. I'm just giving you a hard time. To clarify, I was always better at math and science. We will never play a game of Scrabble. Ever."

Charlotte smiled. "Wise choice. I *am* the queen of Scrabble."

From across the room, Bea let go of another dart. Franco Bellimer said something, prompting Bea to wave her hand at him, a fly to swat away.

One of the women from the corner table snapped her fingers. "Hey, Dana, get me another fork. This one's got, like, grossness on it."

The red-wine drinker's strident voice carried a distinctive, demanding quality that pierced the buzz of background bar noise. The hairs on the back of Charlotte's neck rose to attention.

Shit.

Charlotte looked over. The woman stared back.

The Hickey.

It was hard to tell, with the excess 50 or so pounds, if the woman really was Nicki, Charlotte's second least favorite Biting Walleye. She wore a tight, leather skirt, the pudge of her thighs fighting against the hem like crescent roll dough bursting from its cylindrical packaging. A defining look. The horrors of a well-known cheer uniform. Charlotte didn't have any idea who Nicki's white-wine-drinking buddy was. Nor did she care.

"With you in just a minute, Nicki." Behind the bar, Dana slowly finished polishing the glass in her hands, walked across the room, and plunked down a fresh set of silverware. With Dana's back to Charlotte, the women's heads bent toward each other.

"The Tree?" Nicki's stage whisper carried, a stealthy dagger headed in Charlotte's direction. "I thought that klutzy bitch—"

"Shhh," Dana said, "That's not—"

"Let's get out of here." Charlotte dropped down from her stool and grabbed Jake's hand.

"Oh. Um, sure. Okay."

"I'm ready for that walk." Charlotte pulled him along, but she couldn't resist the urge to take one last look over her shoulder. Nicki laughed—a screech of a sound. She raised her hand and waggled her red-tipped fingers. As if of its own polite accord, Charlotte's free hand slowly waved back.

Dana's cheeks paled. "See you tomorrow, Charlotte?"

"Probably not." Charlotte turned and dragged Jake toward the door.

Bea let fly an effing dart. She gave a whoop as the door of The Surly Sturgeon closed behind Charlotte.

24

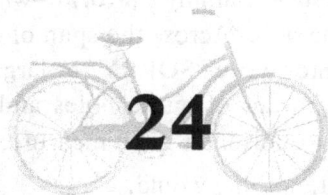

Sammy had continued to ignore Charlotte's numerous sorry messages.

So, she'd upped her game.

Unbeknownst to the little shit, she'd asked Mama Macon to schedule a haircut the Wednesday before Thanksgiving. She didn't care what most of the Lakeside and Marblehead folks thought of her, particularly now that they'd all been reading her life story.

She didn't care about the Danas and the Nickis.

But Sammy? Sammy's opinion of her mattered a great deal. He would forgive her, or she'd have to find a different hairdresser.

And a different best friend.

Charlotte pulled in front of the salon, checked her reflection in the mirror three times, and crept from her car. She grabbed the large cake box from the back seat and leaned against the car door, her eyes drawn to the dim light coming from the interior of The Clip Joint.

What was she so scared of, anyway?

It's just Sammy. Get over yourself.

Taking a deep breath and securing her grip on her box, Charlotte hopped over the welcome mat and teetered in the entrance, once again. Deference? Defiance? She still wasn't sure which.

Definitely, one of those, though.

The bell tinkled a greeting for her eight o'clock appointment, but the front room remained deserted. Charlotte stood at the counter for a few minutes and finally set the cake down. She opened the clear flap. The red velvet—Sammy's favorite—was still intact despite her jump through the door. Across the span of cream cheese icing, she'd had the decorator write "SORRY" as large as possible. She'd added a decorative border of music notes and barber scissors in Miami orange and turquoise, for good measure.

If that didn't do it, nothing would.

Charlotte pulled off her coat, hung it on a rack by the door, and took a seat. She snapped up a women's magazine and flipped through the latest gossip without really registering the content.

A few minutes after eight and no sign of Sammy.

He better not stand her up. She'd wait him out for as long as necessary.

Someone walked past the storefront window, his head a bobbing baseball cap that reminded Charlotte of her father.

8:13 a.m. Still no Sammy.

"Really?" Charlotte ditched the magazine and quickly texted.

Sorry Sorry Sorry Sorry Sorry Sorry Sorry Sorry—

"Come on, Dude." She pressed send and began scrolling through her social media, checking the emails she'd neglected.

8:22 a.m. No Sammy.

Charlotte eyed the curtain separating the front room from the back. Could he just be sitting there? Waiting for her to leave?

"Sammy? You back there?"

He'd have to come to work eventually. Surely, she wasn't the only customer scheduled.

"Sammy? Hey, are you there?"

8:28 a.m. Nothing.

"Come onnnnn, Sammy from Miami, get your ass out here," Charlotte grumbled. She whipped out her phone and put through another text.

Sorry Sorry Sorry Sorry Sorry Sorry Sorry Sorry Sorry—

At exactly 8:30 a.m., a loud bang emanated from the back. Sammy strolled from behind the curtain, juggling a coffee and box of donuts. He plopped the donuts on the reception counter, added a stack of napkins, and set down his coffee without acknowledging Charlotte. He paused, just long enough to read the "Sorry" cake, before shucking his raincoat and throwing it on a hook.

Oh, my gosh.

Charlotte covered her mouth with her hand. They'd time-traveled back a decade. Sammy wore his usual black jeans and red sneakers with a well-worn Billy Joel concert t-shirt from the year they graduated. The cut-off sleeves revealed his sinewy arms peppered with a variety of tattoos. The Marblehead Lighthouse, an addition since they'd matriculated, took up a place of pride on his bicep.

Finally, Sammy spun on his heels to face her and folded his arms across his chest. His lip curled. "Sorry to keep you waiting. How can I help you today? Haircut only?"

Oh. This is going to hurt.

"Yes, please."

"I'm surprised you'd trust a homeboy from Marblehead to do it right. Bet the hairdressers in—Pittsburgh, is it?—are pros at the newest pixie cut." Sammy turned his back on her, motioning for her to follow. "Right this way, miss. Let's get you washed up."

Miss?

Shit. Definitely going to hurt.

It was a good thing Charlotte wasn't getting color or Sammy might dye her purple. Though, in retrospect, perhaps she deserved to let him do his worst, if it would allow him to forgive her.

Sammy ushered Charlotte into the shampoo chair and threw a rolled towel across the back of her neck. Like a bullfighter, he swept a cape into the air, almost slapping Charlotte in the face with it. The drape settled on her chest. He pushed her back into the cradle. She settled into position, and a stream of icy water hit the top of her head.

Charlotte yelped.

"Too cold, miss? One moment."

In seconds, the water went from ice to lava. Eyes watering, Charlotte clenched her teeth, and Sammy plunged his hands under her head, raking his fingers through the strands and soaking her. After a minor adjustment, the water cooled to Goldilocks—just-right.

"Thank you."

A glob of shampoo.

Rinse.

Silence.

A glob of conditioner.

Rinse.

Silence.

Charlotte stared at her best friend from forever. He did not meet her gaze, making the hair-washing process as basic as possible and glancing off to her left, as if watching for someone to walk through the door and save him.

Come on, dude.

Sammy whistled off-key and shoved his fingers deeper into her hair, rubbing and massaging with a little more strength than was absolutely necessary.

"Oh, that feels fantastic." Charlotte smiled.

She gazed up. He scowled down. Massaged harder. Faster.

"Wonderful, Sammy. Just great."

Sammy rolled his eyes up to the fluorescent light filtering through the turquoise fabric draped to set the mood. A swag of orange fringe swung from the corners.

"Love what you've done with the place," Charlotte said. "Very Miami retro."

Sammy turned off the water, dropped a towel on Charlotte's head, and rubbed vigorously. Very, very vigorously.

He hustled back to his station. She scurried to follow and sat, allowing him to whirl her around to greet the mirror. Charlotte snorted. Her hair stuck out in all directions, and Sammy began running a wide-tooth comb through it, gentler this time.

"What do you want?" His eyes refused to meet hers in the mirror.

For you to be my friend again.

"Clean it up?" Sammy said. "Maybe an inch and a half off? Part to the left?"

"Yes, please."

Sammy glanced into the mirror, pulling each side down to assess the length. He wouldn't meet Charlotte's stare. His gaze faded to the left again, and he grabbed a pair of scissors from the soaking container.

"You've got to talk to me eventually, Sammy. I'm not leaving until you do." Charlotte closed her eyes, just like the first time her friend had sheared off 12 inches of her hair. "And, to clarify, I trust you more than any Pittsburgh hairdresser. I always will, you idiot. I'm sorry. I was stupid. I've missed you, and I was wrong to lose touch. I know that now. You can keep being pissed, but at least I'll know I tried. Or, you could forgive me and we could revisit the whole 'best friends' thing. I'd really like that. I could use a best friend."

Eyes still shut, Charlotte smiled and, knowing he was watching her in the mirror, stuck out her tongue.

"Just promise you won't give me a purple Mohawk."

There was a muffled sound, then a pause.

And a snip.

Snip. Snip.

Charlotte kept her eyes shut, finally relaxing her shoulders and sinking into the chair. The meditative sound of the scissors calmed her, and she gave her locks up to the capable hands of the one and only Sammy from Miami. Minutes passed. He used an electric razor to trim the hairline at her neck and lightly brushed the stray hairs away with a towel. He removed the cape from her shoulders.

"Done," Sammy whispered.

Charlotte opened her eyes. It was a good cut—a little more defined than the last time Sammy had taken his scissors to her. The sides were tighter than she was used to, but he'd left just enough layered waves to frame her face and bring out the length of her dark eyelashes and character of the freckles across her nose.

Clean.

Simple.

Charlotte.

"I love it. Thank you."

Sammy dropped the comb onto the counter. He absently wiped the scissors with a towel.

"Are we okay?" Charlotte waited, pleading with him in the mirror.

A sigh.

"Dammit, Char."

"I'm sorry, Sammy. I mean it. I'm really, really, really, really sorry."

"I gathered that from your texts."

Charlotte nodded. "I'm so—"

"Do you even understand what you should be sorry for?" Eyes downcast, Sammy continued neatening his counter. "When I moved here, I didn't know anyone. I was different, but so were you. We were different together. You were my person." He raised his gaze to meet hers. "You were the reason I came to school. Every. Damned. Day. The only reason."

"Same for me," Charlotte said. "You were my person, too."

"Was I? Then why in the hell did you just drop me like I didn't matter? You left, Char, but that wasn't the problem. You fell off the map. I tried so many times to contact you. And you completely ghosted me. What did I do to deserve that?"

"Nothing. You didn't do anything. It wasn't about you. I just... I was so ready to leave everything behind. You know I was. I felt trapped here. I know that doesn't explain anything. It's not an excuse. It's not. I just needed to move on. And I guess I didn't realize how that would affect you." Charlotte dipped her chin. "I didn't mean to forget you, too. That's—"

"That's *exactly* how it felt." Sammy waved the pair of scissors for emphasis. "All my life I was the small kid. The weird kid. The outsider who traveled north to a frozen lake instead of listening to reggae on some hot-as-hell Florida beach. I prefer showtunes and 80s music. I actually like snow. I never fit in down there, and when we first moved to the peninsula, I didn't think I'd ever fit in here. Hell, most people *still* think I'm gay, just because I'm a loud, male hairdresser with Latin dance moves. You were literally my opposite, Char. Pale and tall and awkward and quiet. I thought that was awesome. We were made for each other. Yin and Yang. And I thought you'd understand how alone I felt, because no one else would. I thought you needed me as much as I needed you."

"I did." Charlotte pinched the bridge of her nose. He was confusing her. "I'm sorry if—"

"Jesus, Char. No. Don't you get it? I didn't want you to be my girlfriend. It was never that. I just needed you to be my friend."

"I was," Charlotte said. "I was always your friend. Your best friend."

"Only until you could move on to something better. Until *you* didn't need *me* anymore." Sammy carefully laid the scissors down on the counter. "That's not a best friend."

"Oh, Sammy, no." A wrench in Charlotte's gut doubled her over. She dropped her face in her hands. "That's not true." A shudder ran through her, and she looked up at him, swiping the tears from her cheeks. "How could you think that? I needed you. I will *always* need you. You know me better than anyone. I'll be married for 50 years to some dude I haven't even met yet, and you'll still know me better. Please, Sammy. I was wrong. I'm so, so sorry."

Frowning, Sammy looked back at her. Charlotte scanned the hurt in his eyes. It was done. She'd lost him, for good. And she only had herself to blame. She'd been a terrible friend—not the kind of friend anyone deserved.

Certainly not Sammy.

He turned toward the back room.

"Please, don't go," Charlotte pleaded, watching his reflection in the mirror.

He paused and finally turned.

"Oh, for God's sake." Groaning, he spanned the short distance between them. He wrapped his arms around her from behind, resting his crossed forearms just below her chin, and laid his own chin on the top of her head. "You're stupid. We're stupid. Really, really stupid."

A slow smile split his face, finally, revealing his perfect white teeth against dark skin. His hair was as black as hers, but slightly curlier and longer. It fell over his forehead in a rakish swoosh. If it weren't for her pale features, they could have been siblings.

"You forgive me?" Charlotte's gaze sought Sammy's in the mirror. She placed her hands over his, clenching his fingers beneath hers. "Please, say you forgive me."

"Fine. I forgive you. Just stop with the texting or I'll change my phone number."

"Oh, Sammy."

"Welcome home, Char. It's about damned time."

"Should we cut the cake? It's red velvet."

"'Kay." Sammy smiled. "I'll get some plates."

25

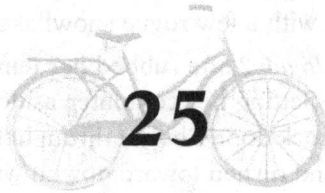

On Thanksgiving Day, Charlotte woke with the beginnings of a headache. The community potluck, starting at three o'clock sharp, would offer a holiday celebration for the year-round residents and a farewell party for many of the seasonal cottage owners who disappeared for the winter to homes in all corners of Ohio, Pennsylvania, Michigan, and beyond. Like it or not, Charlotte expected to bump into someone.

Probably *many* someones.

The regulars who didn't know about her homecoming through the grapevine would be surprised. And with surprises came questions.

Questions about life in Pittsburgh.

Questions about why she hadn't returned since graduation.

Questions about Chuck's wellbeing and the failing business, said in an aside when her dad wasn't paying attention.

She didn't want any of it.

Downstairs, Charlotte found her father asleep in his recliner. In the background, Rockettes high-kicked their way through the

Thanksgiving Day Parade streaming on the television. Adam wasn't up yet, and Charlotte was glad to let him sleep. He had spent his previous evening helping her clean the house, a chore she suspected hadn't been done in months.

Charlotte pulled her laptop from her bag and answered her emails while Chuck slept. On the television, an enormous inflatable dog float dragged tiny humans along on the end of its leash. From the couch, Charlotte spied the lake through the window. It was a windy, overcast day, with a few rogue snowflakes fluttering by.

The first snow? Already? She rubbed her temples. Maybe a walk would do her good. Setting her computer aside, she pulled on her coat and left via the back door. She cut through the parking lot of the bicycle rental shop and turned toward downtown. A few year-round businesses displayed "Black Friday 50% off" signs in their windows, and "For Sale" signs decorated two commercial buildings and three cottages along her path. The Lakeside real estate market fluctuated widely. Turnover would not be good for her father's business.

Just past the Orchestra Hall theater, Charlotte veered left into the park and past the shuffleboard courts. A light glimmered in the window of a small cottage bordering the park, but otherwise she saw no signs of human life. The smell of damp leaves and pine wrapped her in nostalgia. Lakeside touted itself as a bustling vacationer's dream spot in the summer, with laughing children, the *clack, clack, clack* of shuffleboard tournaments, and rowdy teens at the basketball court. But now? It was just Charlotte and deserted streets and the lake.

As she approached the waterfront pavilion, the wind picked up, sending a chill racing along her flesh. With nearly numb fingers, she pulled her hood tighter around her ears. The air on her cheeks woke her more fully than any caffeine could have, and the headache she'd begun the day with swept away with the breeze. The familiar "Dock Closed" warning sign spanned the pavilion entrance, and a spray of whitecaps shot up and over the cement, less than 30 feet away.

A beautiful, raw thing.

Charlotte pulled out her phone and took some video. There was no match for Mother Nature.

And though her father would be even less of a match for the Alzheimer's slowly destroying his mind, all that had happened in the weeks since her return suddenly turned to nothing. She'd get through it, somehow. Charlotte's tension melted away with every howl of the wind, every screech of the gulls, every wall of water meeting the dock.

"Happy Thanksgiving, Lake Erie." She lifted her chin, letting the wind whip her hood away from her face and whisk her sentiment out into open water.

When she returned to Sutton's Choice, Chuck was still sleeping with the parade playing in the background. Before showering, Charlotte tapped on Adam's door.

"About time to get up, kid," she said. "Potluck in a few hours."

A grumble.

She took it as an affirmative.

*   *   *   *   *

Charlotte circled the old, south auditorium twice before finding an open spot.

"For fool's sake, they've *got* to do something about the lack of parking. Crowded as all hell," Bea said. "There had better be a piece of rhubarb pie left, too, or I'm goin' home. That's for damn sure."

"They aren't serving rhubarb this year," Chuck said. "Get out and start walking, old woman."

"Bullshit."

Charlotte glanced at her father in the passenger's seat. He winked.

"Right. Everybody out," Charlotte said, with a wink of her own. *Maybe* they'd have a good day—something to be thankful for.

Adam arrived on the Rusty Banana and swung the bike into a nearby rack just as Charlotte popped the trunk.

"Thanks for giving up your seat in the car," she said. "Can't believe you're still riding that old thing."

"Vintage wheels, man," Adam said.

"Quite."

Jake lifted out the crockpot with Chuck's favorite grape-jelly-coated meatballs, and Charlotte handed Adam a container of chocolate crinkle cookies.

Jake nodded at the remaining pie box. "Rhubarb. Just for you, Bea. Didn't really think we'd expect you to go without dessert, did ya'?"

"You're a good boy, Jakey. Drinks on me after this damned nonsense," Bea said. "God knows, I thought about bringing a flask of vodka for the punch."

"They'd throw you out on your ear," Chuck said. "Lakeside's been dry for more than a century. I doubt that'll change this Thanksgiving."

"Why do you think I opted to run a dive bar within stumbling distance right outside the pearly gates?" Bea chuckled. "Easy money. You've spent a dime or two there yourself, Good-time."

Chuck smiled and led the way, opening the front doors of the building.

Charlotte let everyone else enter and fell in behind Adam. Would she be welcome? Or shamed? Either way, the black sheep of the family had returned to its weird, little, dysfunctional flock. She was still the odd one out. Still The Tree.

Charlotte grimaced. "Nothing to see here, folks."

"What?" Adam turned.

"Nothing."

Just looking for one good day.

And maybe a wishbone.

The woman at the reception desk wore garish makeup, and, hope beyond hope, Sammy hadn't done the dye job on her berry-red hair. Berry Lady's mustard leggings under an orange, cable-knit tunic, a harvest-patterned scarf, and suede boots completed the holiday ensemble.

"Chuck, so glad you could make it." She reached across the table and hugged him. He allowed her to peck his cheek and slyly wiped the lipstick stain away with the back of his hand after she retreated.

A good day.

Chuck hesitated slightly. "Good to see you... Susan."

"Thanks for dropping off the buns yesterday, Bea," Susan said. "It made it easier during set up. So, who else do we have here? Adam, right?"

Adam nodded.

"You look so much like your dad—handsome, of course."

"Um, thanks," Adam said.

Susan eyed Jake up one side and down the other. He held out a hand.

"Jake Forrester. I work over at the marina and do whatever Bea tells me."

"Nice to meet you. That's a smart way to stay on her good side, I'd say." Berry Lady threw Jake a flirtatious smile, and she grasped his hand a might too long.

Charlotte wrinkled her nose. *Really?* The woman was old enough to be his mother.

Chuck shifted from one foot to the other. Charlotte stepped forward.

"Hi. I'm Charlotte, Chuck's daughter."

"Charlie," Chuck said, a beat behind.

Charlotte noticed slight confusion in her father's eyes.

Not a good day?

"I should have known. You're the image of him, too." Susan's gaze traveled from Charlotte to Chuck to Adam. "My goodness. No questioning the Sutton genes."

"Yeah. I suppose not." Charlotte nudged Jake to lead the way. "Let's find Mr. B."

Three long lines of tables spanned the center of the space large enough for a basketball court. Tables burgeoning with the

Thanksgiving potluck offerings of the dozens of people milling about fronted a raised stage at the south end of the room. The walls needed a good scraping and a fresh coat of paint, and a slight musty smell tickled Charlotte's nose as she took a deep breath. She smiled. Nothing had changed, not even the ancient, plastic pumpkin centerpieces on every table.

"There he is." Jake motioned to Franco Bellimer, sitting alone at a long table near the front.

"Lecherous ol' fool saved us a good spot," Bea said.

Jake and Charlotte laughed.

Bea frowned. "What's so funny?"

"Not a blessed thing," Charlotte said.

The group's trek through the room took an eternity.

"Hey, Chuck, loved that story you did about the history of the lighthouse," a woman hollered from a nearby table.

"Thanks," Chuck said.

"What ya think about the Toledo Mud Hens this year?" another voice said behind Charlotte. "Signed a new pitcher. Young guy from Florida."

"We've got the games on at the bar, Frank," Bea said. "You haven't been for a beer in a while. Carolyn keeping you home?"

"Carolyn ain't keepin' me nothin.' She been sleepin' with Davie Smith. We're through, didn't ya' hear?"

"Well, for eff's sake. No, I hadn't. Dammit."

"About them Mud Hens," Frank said. "What ya' think, Chuck?"

"I'm... I'm not sure," Chuck said. "I just don't know this year. S... sorry."

Every few feet, someone stopped them. Bea did most of the talking. Chuck became quieter with each greeting, and Charlotte jumped in to cover her father's inability to remember names and faces. The charismatic man who had always owned the room struggled as the Alzheimer's took that away from him with every step.

A young woman stood up from the nearest table. "Hey, Chuck, can I talk to you about my advertising next week?"

"I'm sorry," Chuck said. "You... you are—"

"Kelly from One Step Up." The woman glanced at Charlotte. "The shoe store in Marblehead. I've used the same ad for the past three years. I want to change things up a bit."

"Sure," Chuck mumbled.

The woman nodded and cocked her head.

"We'll put you on our graphic designer's schedule," Charlotte said. "Just give a call to the office on Monday. Thanks so very much for your business."

"No problem," Kelly said.

Chuck gazed off to the left. "Thank you."

Charlotte had always envied her father's easy camaraderie and ability to befriend anyone, anywhere, a skill she herself did not possess. Putting people at ease was what her father now lacked. This Chuck? This wasn't the real Chuck. This was a shadow of Chuck. Blinking back tears, Charlotte kept her eyes trained on the back of Adam's head.

"Happy Thanksgiving." Franco Bellimer stood up to greet them. "About time. I was afraid if you were any longer, I'd have to lie down on the table to claim our space. I didn't have enough coats to hold our chairs, and the vultures were circling."

"Cripes. Relax." Bea chuckled. "Odds are, we're the only ones who want to sit with the likes of you."

"Fine by me." Franco pulled out the chair beside him and practically forced Bea into it. "You're all I need, love."

"Hey, guys." Sammy waved from several tables over. "Whoop! Whoop! Char's in da' house." Nearby voices stuttered to a buzz.

"You're joining us, aren't you?" Charlotte motioned for the Macons to grab a chair.

"How's the haircut?" Sammy plopped down across from Charlotte. "Working okay? If those bangs give you any trouble, come in and I can take care of them." He nodded in Jake's direction and reached his hand across the table. "I'm Sammy Macon, and this is Mama."

"Jake Forrester." Jake smiled and shook Sammy's hand.

"Nice to meet you, Jake," Mama Macon said. "Any friend of Charlotte's is a friend of ours."

"Likewise," Jake said.

"'Kay. So, Char told me you've been helping with things." Sammy's gaze shifted to Charlotte's father.

"When I can," Jake said. "You're the friend who chopped off Charlotte's hair, right? Pretty funny story."

"A riot. I thought Char's mom was going to kill me."

"I can imagine." Jake smiled. "I'm surprised we haven't met before, at the bar or something."

Sammy shrugged. "To be honest, I'm too busy to do much else but work. With the holidays, I've barely made it out of my shop. I own The Clip Joint salon. Crazy busy this time of year."

"Clever name."

"Thanks. It was either that or The Blow Job." Sammy mimed drying his hair with a wicked grin. "I didn't think that would go over as well with the locals, and since most of them already think I'm the gay hairdresser, that would have all but settled it."

"The Clip Joint has its own infamy, son," Franco said.

Sammy's brows arched. "Yeah. I was thinking about putting in a rooftop Mary Jane garden this summer. On the hush-hush. Maybe offer a little muscle relaxer to my clients to make the hair-cutting experience more enjoyable."

"Oh, Sammy." Charlotte shook her head.

"There's a market for everything, I suppose." Franco cleared his throat and reached an arm around Bea's shoulder. "Sure are lookin' good this fine afternoon, woman." He gave her shoulder a squeeze. "Smelling good, too. Is that a new perfume?"

"It's liniment, you fool." Bea plucked Franco's hand from her shoulder and dropped it, none too gently, on the table. "My joints are aching. Gonna snow soon, for damn sure. I can feel it."

Charlotte and Jake exchanged a look.

"So glad you stayed, sweet Charlotte," Mama Macon said. "Sammy finally smiles again. He smiles and smiles."

"Thanks, Mama." Charlotte glanced at Chuck. Lost to the conversation, he gazed off into the distance as if he were a million miles away. "I've still got to go back to Pittsburgh soon. Just getting things organized first."

"But when are you and Sammy giving me grandchildren, dear girl? You're in the prime of life."

Charlotte closed her eyes. "Oh, Mama—"

"Grandchildren?" Jake asked.

"Of course," Mama Macon said. "Lots and lots of them. My Sammy and Charlotte will make beautiful babies, don't you think?"

"Yep." Jake's eyes locked with Charlotte's. "Charlotte would definitely make beautiful babies."

Sammy snorted and shifted in his chair. "Wouldn't she?"

Heat crept up Charlotte's neck. "I'm not ready for children. I'm not even married."

"That can be arranged." Mama reached her hand across the table and patted Charlotte's. "We'll talk at dinner next week. Won't we?"

"'Kay, Mama, let it go," Sammy said. "Char and I aren't getting married."

"But you'd make such a beautiful couple," Mama said.

"We're just friends," Charlotte said. "Best friends."

"That's about as much as I can handle," Sammy said.

Amused, Charlotte shook her head. Mama Macon still wanted little Charlotte and Sammy grandchildren—Chammies, as Sammy had dubbed their imaginary offspring—after so much time had passed. Mama had married them off to each other since their first Homecoming dance back in their freshman year, when Sammy was still considered new to town and Charlotte was The Tree, without any grace or social skills.

The two of them made an awkward Homecoming pair. Charlotte towered above Sammy's 5'2" frame and took to standing perfectly still while he danced circles around her—his hips undulating to the cha-cha, merengue, salsa, or whatever Latin dance moved him. It mattered not what song the DJ was playing—fast, slow, or somewhere in between. Sammy danced with abandon, with a complete lack of concern for onlookers and what anyone was whispering behind their palms. He'd made her howl with laughter on a night that could have been miserable. Likely would have been. Of course, the Danas, the Nickis, and the Mike McKenzies laughed right along with them—at them. But Sammy's policy had been to laugh first, so it wouldn't hurt when others joined in. It was a good policy. Charlotte had pretty much lived that same policy ever since.

From the safety of her chair, she finally took a moment to scan the other tables. Most of the attendees were Chuck's age and older, but Charlotte spotted several from her generation. In the far corner, one of the Baker twins—Lauren or Larissa—played carols on an old baby grand piano. Charlotte had never known either of them well, only seen them perform. Identical, they not only looked alike—blonde sticks with green eyes—but participated in band, choir, and every show at the local community theater. During senior year, the Baker twins had announced they would go off to New York City to find their destiny on the Broadway stage. Maybe only one twin had succeeded, and this—playing Christmas carols at a potluck in Lakeside, Ohio—was the destiny of the other. She wasn't sure who'd gotten the better deal.

At the drinks station, Dana lifted her daughter Trinity and allowed the little girl to raise the ladle and pour some punch into a clear, plastic cup. Only about half the liquid made it to its destination. Dana acknowledged Charlotte with a nod and a smile, before walking over to talk to Kate Fallow, who stood in a far corner with her arm around the waist of a thin woman with short hair, presumably her partner Rachel. Off in another corner, Mrs. T sat with Snuggles nestled in a bag on her shoulder.

"I'm going to grab a drink," Charlotte said, standing. "Dad, can I get you anything? Bea? Anyone?"

"I'll help," Adam said.

After taking orders, they headed off to the punch table. Charlotte kept her head down and passed a pair of Biting Walleyes grads wearing too much makeup and way too little clothing. Charlotte's classmates stopped their chattering.

"Hi, Charlotte."

"Heard you were—"

"Hey." Charlotte gave them a single nod of acknowledgment but sped up. They hadn't given her the time of day back in high school. Now was not the time to start. With Adam, her silent shadow, she passed a basketball player and his family and a teacher Charlotte had never had in class. At the drinks table, she eyed the punch. A fabricated mint green, it looked like the classic combination of ginger soda and sherbet ice cream—the same punch served at every potluck since the beginning of time. She lifted a cup to her lips and let the foam form a mustache on her upper lip, the sticky sweetness tasting like the nectar of gods.

She and Adam poured drinks and turned to trek back to the table.

But Nicki and a mini carbon copy stood in the way.

"Well, look who's still standing, sweetie."

Shit.

Nicki's smile didn't reach her eyes. The woman scanned Charlotte's body from head to toes and back up again.

"Nicki." Charlotte ran the back of her hand across her mouth. The Hickey and her daughter, about eight years old, wore matching leaf-patterned leggings and olive sweaters with fuzzy, brown boots. They wore matching lip gloss. They wore matching gold-hoop earrings. Nicki's dyed hair was the exact blonde shade as her daughter's. If Charlotte didn't know better, she'd have thought the pair could give Lauren and Larissa Baker some competition.

Nicki placed her hand on her daughter's shoulder. "Shanna, this is The Tree. The Tree, my daughter Shanna."

Shit. Shit. Shit.

"Why's she called The Tree, Mom?" The girl's strident, whiny voice mimicked her mother's.

Why? Why, indeed.

A murmur from behind. A whisper to the side.

Charlotte kept her eyes down. A quiet settled on their little corner of the room.

Her own heartbeat hammered in her ears.

26

Clenching her teeth, Charlotte offered the child a thin smile. "It's just a nickname."

Nicknames are nothing. Nothing.

"My real name is Charlotte. It's so very nice to meet you, Shanna. You look just like your mom."

"Yes, I do." The little girl flipped a swath of blonde hair behind her shoulder.

Dear God.

"Charlotte and I were friends in high school, sweetie," Nicki said, her voice loud enough to reach the nearby tables. "She's still so tall and skinny. Don't you think she looks a lot like a tree?"

Charlotte swallowed. What do you even say to that?

"Friends?" Adam shook his head. "Man, not likely." As seamless as a knife through butter, he barreled forward and cut through mother and daughter. He motioned over his shoulder at Charlotte. "Dude, better things to do than this. Let's go."

Shaking, Charlotte forced herself forward. It was ridiculous. How could such an awful human—a grown woman—still make her feel like the tree that she was? It wasn't okay. It would never be okay.

Charlotte took a breath and halted in front of Nicki, nearly spilling green punch all over those leafy leggings.

"Adam's right. There *are* far better things to do than be bullied. You haven't changed at all in the past 10 years, have you?"

"What—"

"I'm sorry," Charlotte said. "Really, really sorry."

"Sorry? Sorry for what?" Nicki pulled her daughter close to her side.

Charlotte glanced at the child and weighed her next words. "I'm *sorry* for whatever it is you think I did to you. I must have done something pretty horrible, because you're clearly still not over it." Charlotte planted her feet, a cup in each hand. "So, I apologize. I. Am. Sorry." She swept one of the cups through the air dramatically—gracefully—without spilling a drop. "Let's move on, Nicki." Charlotte forced a smile to her lips and looked down at Shanna. "My mom always told me to treat people how I'd like to be treated."

Nicki's face turned a brilliant shade of red that clashed horribly with her sweater. "Well, I never—"

"Is there a problem, Charlotte?"

Charlotte turned. Dana had returned to the punch table, a look of concern plastered on her beautifully made-up face.

"Nope. Not anymore. Nicki and I were just catching up. Practically like old times."

"I bet." Dana frowned. "I told you to leave her be, Hickey." She squared off with the bigger woman. "What kind of example are you setting for your daughter?"

"A bad one," Adam murmured.

"Mom, what's a hickey?" Shanna said.

Someone laughed at a nearby table. It was time to end it. Whether she was just like Nicki or not, the child didn't deserve to hear about her mother's hickey ways.

"I've got no problem with you, Nicki, but I'm done playing games," Charlotte said quietly. "This needs to stop. Now. You stay out of my way, and I'll stay out of yours."

"Generous offer," Dana said. "You should take her up on it, Nicki."

Charlotte smiled. "Thanks, Dana."

Nicki shifted from one tall boot to the other. Finally, she cleared her throat. "Sorry," she said, not meeting Charlotte's eyes. "I... was just joking."

"We both know that isn't entirely true. But your apology is accepted."

Nicki nodded, her hand reaching for Shanna's.

Charlotte glanced at the young girl who looked so much like her mother. "It was very, very nice meeting you, Shanna." She offered Nicki a pointed look. "Happy Thanksgiving to you both."

"Happy Thanksgiving," Nicki said.

"Drinks on me next time you're at the bar, Charlotte," Dana said. "I believe I owe you at least one. Maybe five."

Charlotte smiled. "I would love that. Let's do dinner some night soon before I go."

"Yes, let's."

"Well, I've got to get back to my dad. See you." Charlotte took the lead back to the table. Everyone sat mute, staring at her.

"You all right, Char?" Sammy said.

"Nothing to see here. Carry on."

"You sure? Couldn't hear everything, but it looked vicious."

Charlotte shrugged. "Yeah, it kinda was. Just a little unfinished business I think I've finally put behind me. Feels pretty good, actually."

Franco Bellimer gave Charlotte a nod.

"You won that round," Adam said. "Hands down."

"There's no winning against Nicki," Charlotte said, "but I really appreciated the back-up. Thanks, Adam."

"Sure. Been there."

"Water over the bridge. Under the bridge. Whatever," Bea said. "Some people aren't worth the toilet paper they wipe their asses with. Shit's all the same."

"What she said," Jake added.

As if in unspoken agreement, everyone started talking again amongst themselves. Charlotte leaned back in her chair and let their voices wash over her like a warm breeze. Her heart thumped. Her head thumped. The incident with Nicki had taken her right back to high school and the many times she'd endured similar incidents.

It was stupid—stupid she could still let it bother her.

Chuck tapped her on the knee. He leaned in and whispered, "You did good. What's past is past, kid. Life is too short."

Charlotte breathed in the comforting smell of her father's after-shave.

What's past is past. "Yeah, Dad, to steal one of your quotes from Yogi Berra, 'It ain't over till it's over.' I sure hope that high school nonsense is over."

Chuck nodded. "Look past the negative and find the positive."

"Cheers to that." Charlotte took a sip of her minty drink.

He was right, in so many ways. The Hickey wasn't worth the energy.

Charlotte's gaze shifted to Jake chatting with the Macons about fishing charters and his algae bloom research. His wool sweater showed the breadth of his shoulders. Even with the beard, Charlotte could tell there was a dimple in his left cheek. He was an easy, positive distraction.

"That's wild," Sammy said. "Marine biology, huh? I've always liked the Marines."

Charlotte choked on her sherbet punch, the liquid trickling down her windpipe.

Jake smiled. "Got to love the Marines."

Chuck hammered his daughter on the back. "Cough it out, Charlie. Cough it out."

"Here, dear." Mama Macon handed Charlotte a napkin.

"You gonna make it?" Sammy said.

"I'm fine. You do know marine biology has nothing to do—"

"Charlotte?"

The lyrical voice was unmistakable. Charlotte turned and jumped to her feet, almost tipping her chair over in the process.

"Jenny." She threw her arms around the tiny Asian woman, who looked just as she'd looked in high school, but nicely pregnant. "I can't believe it."

"I thought it was you. I overheard somebody say The Tree put The Hickey in her place."

"It was about time. Wow, Jenny, you look fantastic." Charlotte's attention shifted to the tall, bearded man by Jenny's side. "Congratulations. So, you two got married? How'd you ever swing that, Grant?"

"I bribed her. I promised season football tickets if she'd go out with me," Grant Warren said.

Jenny shrugged. "It worked. I'm a sucker for Dawgs tickets."

"She's upped the payoff several times, though, over the years. I've had to get us tickets to every other Cleveland team. Plus, we hit at least a couple of Toledo Mud Hens games a year and, of course, there's hockey. Keyboard nerd falls in love with beautiful sports fanatic in small, waterfront town. Sounds like a Christmas movie."

Charlotte chuckled. Grant had barely squeaked out a high tenor in his teens and had been unable to say more than a few words around Jenny. Back then, she'd been more interested in sports than quiet, pimply-chinned Grant, the one guy with a crush bigger than Jenny herself. He'd grown into a man with a lot more to say, apparently, and in a much deeper voice.

"I have a box at the Cleveland baseball stadium," Grant added. "You should all join us sometime. You'd like that, wouldn't you, Chuck? Seeing the old team?"

"What?"

Charlotte gently nudged her father. "To catch a baseball game, Dad."

"Oh." Chuck nodded. "Yes, I don't think I've been to one in years."

"Hot dogs on the house," said Grant. "And beers, too."

"Sounds fun."

Charlotte meant it. She had not been to a game herself in more than two decades. She'd always hated baseball, but, with the right company, maybe that could change.

People *could* change if they wanted. Grant was proof. He'd lost the acne, bought and sold a software empire, and found a clothier to dress him—all for the love of Jenny.

"I'll be in Pittsburgh, but I could drive up to meet you sometime this summer if you don't mind bringing Dad and Adam to the game," Charlotte said. "The Cleveland stadium is what? About halfway between here and Pittsburgh?"

"About," said Grant. "Great, then. I'll set it up."

"So, where *do* you live? Still Lakeside?"

"Grant shook his head. "We moved about a month ago to Catawba Island. Not too far away. Built a house near the golf course so I can take out clients. We do a fair amount of entertaining, and our place in Lakeside just wasn't big enough."

"You ain't movin' the boats this spring, are ya?" Bea said roughly.

"Of course not."

"We've had dockage at Shores Marina for years," Jenny said, in an aside to Charlotte. "Grant has a 32-foot sailboat, but I prefer our motorboat."

"Why?" Charlotte said. "I've always loved to sail."

"Sailing is fine, but it's—"

"Way too slow for my wife," Grant said. "She's an adrenaline junky. It's all about the speed. She'll be early to our own son's birth."

"When are you due?" Bea said.

"The third week of March." Jenny rubbed her stomach lightly. "I'm hoping for a week earlier, so I don't have to give up our March Madness tickets."

"Well, of course," Charlotte said.

Grant placed his hand on Bea's shoulder. "I'd like to talk, if you have the time? Maybe discuss some mutually beneficial business opportunities? I've been looking into investing in waterfront commercial property. Would you ever consider partnering?"

Bea's sparse eyebrows rose. For once, the marina owner had nothing to say, but she offered a slight nod.

"Let's schedule something in the next several weeks," Grant said.

How would this impact the newspaper? Charlotte frowned. It was no secret the marina wasn't doing as well as it should. Bea couldn't afford to put in fancy, heated storage units and dry-dock services many of the new marinas provided for their customers. If Grant was considering buying Bea out, or even investing in the property, it could mean the end of the marina or a whole new beginning.

"We've got room at the table," Franco said. "You folks want to join us?"

"Thanks," Jenny said, "but Grant's family saved us some seats, and I see a couple of potential donors I need to talk to, so we can get the new football stadium built. We hope to break ground in a year, if we can get the funding."

"Sounds like a lot of work." Charlotte turned to her father. "Should we do a story?"

Chuck nodded.

"I saw the article you did on the high school principal," Jenny said. "Nice job, Charlotte."

"Thanks."

"I'm so glad you're back in town," Jenny said. "You were missed around here."

Charlotte smiled. "Maybe we should meet up some night at The Surly Sturgeon. We could talk about the stadium."

Jenny nodded. "Absolutely."

They exchanged phone numbers and Jenny excused herself, her husband trailing behind, like some quiet, business-like bodyguard. It was good to see them. They made an odd but perfect pair.

As attendees got settled in their seats, redheaded Susan scampered up onto the stage.

"Good afternoon, Lakeside." The microphone squealed, and she took a step back from the podium. "Thank you all for coming out on this blustery Thanksgiving. Please wait until we call your table, and we'll get you through the food line as quickly as possible. But first, Rev. Salamon, would you please help us give thanks for the bounty we are soon to receive?"

A stooped gentleman with thin, white hair and a bowler hat shuffled to the stage. Rev. Salamon was the fifth generation of reverends from the Salamon family to bless the Thanksgiving potluck over the years. Every Rev. Salamon Charlotte had ever met was stooped with thin, white hair.

The reverend stopped two feet away from the microphone and removed his hat. Charlotte understood virtually nothing of his mumbled blessing, but raised her voice, sheep-like, to say "Amen."

"Jesus Christ, let's eat," Bea muttered. "I'm damn near starvin'."

Despite Bea's blasphemy, or perhaps because of it, their table was called first.

"After you, love." Franco pulled Bea's chair out for her.

"I'm not some delicate flower, you damned fool."

Charlotte fell into step behind her father. Her stomach grumbled as she approached the food table straining under platters of turkey, vegetable and fruit trays, multiple jello salads of varying degrees of color and chunkiness, green bean casseroles, white and sweet mashed potatoes (the latter of which with obligatory marshmallow topping), seven varieties of stuffing, and three cranberry relishes. The desserts included home-baked cookies and, conservatively, 20 pies, half of which were pumpkin. Charlotte loaded up—heavy on mashed potatoes and stuffing, light on jello salad and cranberry. Returning to the table, she sat down and tucked in.

"Oh. My. Heavens." She plunged her fork into a mound of starch.

Chuck gave her a pat. "Slow down, Charlie. You'll make yourself sick."

"I'm not five, Dad."

Chuck shrugged. "Alzheimer's or no, I can still play the father."

Fighting the urge to refute the comment, Charlotte squeezed her father's hand. "Yes. Yes, you can." She glanced across the table at Jake, her gaze passing to Adam and Chuck and Sammy and Mama Macon. She felt lighter, in that moment, happier than she'd expected to. Even dealing with The Hickey had lifted her spirits.

Franco raised his glass. "I'd like to propose a toast."

Everyone raised their glasses.

"To family and friends... and friends that are family."

"Hear, hear." Bea tilted her cup to Bellimer's.

Hear, hear.

Charlotte tipped her own drink toward her father's. "Happy Thanksgiving."

A chorus of responses fired from the table, and everyone returned to their plates. Charlotte paused, again looking around the room.

The blond twin at the piano, Lauren or Larissa, began a spirited rendition of "Silent Night," causing her plate of food to bounce on the edge of the piano. Dana and her daughter shared a giggle. Grant's arm rested on the back of Jenny's chair, their heads inches apart. Berry-red Susan stood near the food table, unnecessarily directing people to take a plate before proceeding through the line. Like his parting shot at the end of a church service, Rev. Salamon shook hands with each Lakesider and offered a "Peace be with you."

Taking a bite of stuffing, Charlotte glanced at her father. Chuck's gaze flitted from one corner of the room to the other.

Taking it all in—

The squeal of metal chairs being pushed back from tables.

Children's laughter.

Neighborly chatter.

Not so "Silent Night."

It was unreal. The Lakeside persona of a porch community with good people living side-by-side next to good people offered a life-size display in the oversized, drafty, old building with drab paint and berry-red Susan.

The Hickeys didn't matter. Not in that moment.

The buzz rose to a fever pitch, sending energy pulsing through the room. Charlotte glanced again at her father. Chuck glared at the twin at the piano, his fork lifted partially to his mouth.

"Who is that?"

"What?"

Chuck slowly spun his loaded utensil, allowing the food to drop back onto the plate with a splatter. His hand tremored as he stared at the bare fork. He thrust it at the piano player.

"Who is that?" Chuck's voice sounded agitated, angry. "Is this... mine?"

Charlotte's father's brain—working so hard for the past hour keeping up with the names and the "Hi, Chucks" and the noise, noise, noise—had suddenly had enough.

Charlotte pushed her plate away. The moment sat frozen in her mind, ready to replay over and over.

"Can I help you, Dad?"

Chuck ducked his head. Charlotte placed her fingers over her father's and loaded another forkful. She inched his hand to his mouth and gathered his napkin, dabbing at the corners of his lips after he swallowed. The look of terror in Chuck's eyes almost broke her.

She still knew so little about her father's health.

She knew little about the future. And Adam. And returning to small-town Ohio.

What *did* she know?

The disease was progressing. She was trapped at the highest peak of a rollercoaster of responsibility, with no hope of getting off before the plummet. She had choices to make.

And time was slipping away.
That's what she knew.

27

MIDDLE SCHOOL

The front door slammed, the bark of wood reverberating throughout the house. Fourteen-year-old Charlotte heard it and *felt* it through the cottage's paper-thin walls.

"He's a dead man!"

Hearing her mother's outburst from the floor below, Charlotte decided to stay out of the way until the anger blew over like a 60-second Northeaster, as it usually did. She rolled over on her bed and stared at the ceiling. A cobweb fluttered in a corner of the wood beams.

One Mississippi.

Two Mississippi.

"I do everything around here," Elise yelled, at no one in particular. "And the shit's off having a good time."

Charlotte reached below and grabbed her journal from under her mattress, jumped from her bed, snagged a pencil from her desk, and exited onto the upper-level porch. She slumped down in the rocker and pulled her hoodie up to block out the noise.

The lake was unusually flat, the water gently lapping at the rocks at the water's edge. On the cool, spring day, the tufts of white from the nearby cottonwoods drifted like snow along the path. Several boats dotted the water. It would be just a couple of weeks before the lake was littered with them.

At the marina, a familiar figure wandered into view and opened the gate leading from The Surly Sturgeon. Until Memorial Day, the much-used entrance remained unlocked, a convenience for the Suttons as they came and went from the marina.

Mom would say it was *too* convenient for Chuck, who spent more time at the bar with Bea and over at Put-in-Bay or on Kelleys Island every Saturday night. Charlotte's mother stayed home with her daughter. She took Charlotte to every team practice. She put food on the table and washed all of Charlotte's uniforms. She did do "everything." Chuck spent as much time as possible away from the house. Mom spent as much time as possible making up for Chuck.

Do either of them even want me around?

Chuck weaved a bit, methodically placing his steps. He'd probably had too much to drink. Mom would be pissed.

Charlotte sighed. They were exhausting, and it wouldn't be a fun night for anyone.

Chuck came closer, whistling a familiar, but not truly distinguishable, tune. Suddenly, her mother hurtled out the cottage door. It slammed back with a thump that, again, reverberated beneath Charlotte's feet.

"Dammit, Chuck." Elise's blond hair whipped about her shoulders in waves. "Where the hell you been? Supposed to go for a girls' night at the winery. You're late."

"Easy, El." Chuck slurred his words and almost tumbled from the path. "I'm here now. You can still go."

"You're drunk."

"I'm not. Go, El. I got this."

Charlotte watched from above.

"Shit, Chuck. I do all the cooking. I clean and take Charlotte to all her practices." Elise's fists rested on her hips, her shoulders back. "It's overwhelming. I just wanted this one night. Some 'me' time."

Charlotte pulled her knees up to her chin and wrapped her arms around her legs.

"You go off and do whatever you damn well please," Elise said. "I don't get to. Charlotte's our responsibility. You know what one of those is? A responsibility? She's yours and mine, not just mine."

"Sorry." Chuck listed a bit to port, as if he'd roll down the waterfront path along with the cottonwood fluff.

Elise crossed her arms. "What's so damned hard? Huh?"

"I'll take over the rest of the night," Chuck said. "Charlie and I can go get ice cream and maybe play a round of shuffleboard. It'll be fun. You go out with your girlfriends."

"Just like you go out with *your* girlfriends?" Elise said.

Chuck stilled.

"You think I'm stupid, Chuck? I know what you're up to when you go off to the islands. I know why you have the boat, and I know why you never ask me to go with you."

"Wrong," Chuck said. "You're wrong, El. You know nothing."

"I'm tired of this shit, Chuck."

Charlotte shifted, holding the rocker as steady as possible so no motion from above would give away her position. If they saw her listening, they'd want to talk to her about it.

That would only make things worse.

Her mother had said for years that Good-time Charlie was out looking for a good time, one that his own wife and daughter couldn't provide. Her mother had made other comments, in private, but this was the first time Charlotte had known her parents to fight openly about it. It was a very small community. Even in the off-season, the gossip chain could get the rumor out—about everything and everyone—faster than facts could circulate. Lights shown in the cottage to her left. Old Mrs. Branniger lay on her wicker chaise, listening just as intently to Chuck and Elise. If Chuck was really looking for a good time, the rest of Lakeside would know it now, too.

Swiping a tear from her cheek, Charlotte left her parents to argue on the lawn. She stuffed her journal under her mattress, curled up on her bed, and pulled her threadbare Yogi Bear-a to her chin. She hated all the fighting and her father's empty chair at the dinner table.

Elise was tired of this shit.

But Charlotte was, too.

28

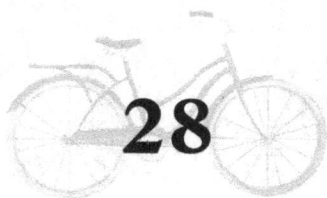

"You're not coming back until after New Year's?" Elliot said. "But I was going to take you somewhere special for Christmas. I already have reservations."

Parked in front of Stanner's Hardware, Charlotte tapped her fingers on the wheel. She peered down the street. She could just barely make out the The Clip Joint sign. Maybe after her appointment, she could take Sammy to lunch.

"I'm sorry." She checked her phone. "Look, Elliot, thanks for checking in, but I've got to go. I've got a meeting in less than five minutes."

Short of simply hanging up, she didn't know how to get her ex-boyfriend to take the hint. When, and how, she'd given him the misguided idea they'd spend the holiday together, she had no idea. He was blind to the reality of their relationship.

Or lack thereof.

Elliot sighed. "Does Tania know—"

"Of course, she knows. I'm working remotely. My father isn't well, Elliot. I can hardly leave him right now."

"Sure. Sure. I completely understand. You want me to come up there for Christmas? I'd love to meet your dad. I'll take some days off. It's okay if I bring Alfredo, right? He doesn't do very well in the car, though."

"Elliot—"

"What is it? About a three-hour drive? I'll have to give him some sleepy pills, or he'll throw up. What about gifts? You'll have to send me a list of who I should buy for. Are there any restaurants open on New Year's Eve?"

"Elliot—"

"I *have* to take you out on New Year's Eve. Somewhere special."

Dear God, make it stop.

"Elliot!" Charlotte took a deep breath. "I'm sorry. We. Are. Not. Dating. We haven't been for months. We already tried that, remember? I think it's best if we see other people. Besides, I need to concentrate on my dad right now."

"But, Charlotte—"

"Please. Don't. Let's keep this professional from now on, okay? And, um, Happy New Year. Give Alfredo a hug for me."

Charlotte hung up. The weight on her chest fell away like a feather. It was finally done. Her only regret was how awkward it would be returning to the Pittsburgh office. Even more so living in the condo down the hall. She'd figure that out later.

Charlotte turned off the engine, took another cleansing breath, and got out of the car. Holding her father's old leather portfolio tight to her chest, she swiped her sweaty palm down the length of her pants and pushed a smile to her lips.

She stepped into Stanner's Hardware, and Jim looked up from the counter. "Well, hey, Charlie, what's up? I heard you were still here. We haven't gone for that drink yet, have we?"

"No, I guess we haven't."

"Need to catch a football game." Jim pointed to his furry brown and orange hat with plush dog ears hanging down on each side of

221

his head. "Woof, woof. Go, Dawgs."

"Nice. Yeah, I've been pretty busy. I decided to stay through the holidays, though, and help out Dad."

"That's great. How is Chuck?"

"Okay. He could be better." Charlotte shrugged. "Speaking of dads, is yours around? I have an appointment to talk about advertising."

"Sure thing. Let me get him for you."

Jim went into the back room, leaving Charlotte with her nerves and portfolio. A few moments later, Randy Stanner emerged, his cane tap, tap, tapping on the wood-slatted floor.

"Great to see you, young lady."

"Hi, Mr. Stanner. Still have the time to talk about the newspaper? I'm trying to help Dad bring on some new advertisers before I take off in January."

Randy's bushy eyebrows rose an inch. "You're really going back to Pittsburgh, huh?" He motioned for her to follow him. "Anything we can do to help, child. Come on into the back, and, for the love of all that is holy, call me Randy. Mr. Stanner sounds like some old fart."

"Thanks, Randy." Charlotte inched past the portly man and into a windowless room with wall-to-wall beige filing cabinets and a mid century desk spanning more than half of the small space. She sat down on the corner of a chair overflowing with invoices.

"Sorry, let me get that for you." Randy shuffled over and transported the papers to a bigger pile on top of a nearby cabinet.

Charlotte scanned the office. Leaning towers of boxes looked like they'd sprouted, weed-like, out of the floors and walls. On Randy's desk sat a coffee can spilling over with screws and nails. Random plumbing pipes—the elbows and oblong tubes of white looking much like a jumbled pile of oversized pasta—littered one corner, and an elaborate clock made from welded-together machinery gears graced the space above Stanner's desk.

Randy sat down and just as quickly popped back up again. "One second." He poked his head out the door. "Heads up, Jimmy. Little Dana McKenzie is supposed to be here soon about that part-time office job. Entertain her until I can finish up with Charlie. We'll just be a minute."

"Dana is looking for a job?" Charlotte said.

Randy shrugged. "More like we're looking for an employee. I asked her to stop by. With her working nights at the bar, I thought she might like some steady daylight hours during the week, now that her little girl is going to school." Randy swept his hand through the air. "We don't need someone full-time, but we're a bit behind on our paperwork. What we need is someone who is organized, and Dana's certainly that. I think she could use the extra hours during the off-season, when the bar slows down."

"Sounds like a great fit."

"That family sure has had a time of it." Randy scratched the acne scars on his cheek. "So, then, let's get down to it. You're trying to sell some ads for the newspaper, huh?"

Charlotte blew out the breath she'd been holding. "Yes. Would you be interested?"

"Well, we haven't done much print advertising the past few years. Haven't really needed it, being in business for so long. Most of our clients come through referrals from neighbors."

Charlotte nodded. "I understand, but I've actually been working on adding digital advertising. Starting in January, the newspaper will offer businesses the opportunity to advertise on Chuck's website and include a direct link back to their own websites. We'll be pushing advertisers out on social media, as well. The new blog page I'm setting up will include all of Dad's essays. They're very popular, and I'm going to be writing for it, as well. Digital ads could be a great way to draw in some new people beyond Lakeside and Marblehead. Our readership covers three counties."

"Huh," Randy said. "Well, I sure do love a Sutton story. Your timing isn't half bad, either. Part of the reason we're hiring is because

Jimmy is breaking in another store. We've been renovating a place in Sandusky."

"Oh, you'll definitely want to advertise that." Charlotte laid an ad sheet on the desk. "If you look here, we expect the newspaper's website to produce a significant jump in traffic. Every advertiser who purchases space on the site will also receive a feature article in a print issue of your choice. The new Stanner store would make a really great story."

"Sold," Randy said. "Sounds like a right fine idea you got there, Charlie. I'll retire sooner than later, and Jimmy has big plans. Got to stay up with the times, I reckon, and if us helping you will help us too, well, why not?"

"Thanks, Randy."

"Always glad to do business with a friend." Stanner's hand engulfed Charlotte's. "That's what we're here for. Call me sometime next week, and we'll schedule a proper meeting to discuss the details."

"Great." Charlotte stood up just as the exterior door slammed.

"That must be Dana," Randy said. "Impeccable timing."

They returned to the front. Dana stood next to Jim, and they peered down at her phone. The top of her head came to well below his chin.

"Hey," Charlotte said.

Dana glanced up and smiled. Jim continued looking over her shoulder.

"Man, Trinity looks just like you," he said. "Check it out, Charlotte. Doesn't she look like a blond copy of her mama?"

Charlotte leaned in. Trinity, in a head-to-toe bunny costume, grinned at the camera. Her front tooth was missing, adding to the look. She carried a huge bucket of Halloween candy.

"Cute. A mini-Dana, for sure. Except the eyes," Charlotte said. "Those are definitely Mike's."

Dana nodded. "You're right. Mike had the best eyes."

"So, the Stanners want to put you to work?"

"We'd be lucky to have her." Jim transferred his weight from one foot to the other. His cheeks reddened. "Sure could use your help in the office, Dana. Sure could."

"But I don't have any office experience." Dana shrugged. "To be honest, I'm not sure how helpful I would be."

"I think you'd be real helpful," Jim said. "I'll teach you."

"You're plenty smart enough, girl," Randy said, "and a very hard worker. That's all we're looking for."

Indecision flooded Dana's face.

"You'd be perfect," Charlotte said, nudging her.

"Oh, I don't know—"

"You should do it, Dana. You've got this."

"You really think so?"

"I do." Charlotte sidled toward the entrance. "Well, thanks again, Randy. I don't want to take up any more of your time. We'll talk next week."

Randy came from around the counter and offered one more handshake. "No problem at all. Anything for a friend."

"See ya." Charlotte opened the door.

"Bye, Charlotte," Dana said.

"Later." Jim shook his head, throwing dog ears left and right. He grinned and quickly returned his attention to Dana.

Charlotte settled into her car but didn't turn on the ignition right away. An almost giddy laugh burst from her lips. She'd done it. She'd sold advertising for her father's paper. And it hadn't been hard. Easy, even.

Smiling, she gave Chuck's old portfolio a pat, set it on the seat beside her, and turned toward home.

* * * * *

Later that afternoon, Charlotte emailed the ad agency her most recent project. The holiday ads would be back to her for edits by the end of the day. She liked writing remotely and had worked surprisingly fast, sitting at her desk in the upstairs bedroom with the old dollhouse, old Yogi Bear-a, and old memories. Rather than looking out at the Allegheny River, though, her office had a view of Lake Erie, a sight that would never, ever grow dull.

Finishing for the day, Charlotte shut down her computer and wandered downstairs. Her father was asleep in his recliner, a blanket tucked around his legs and the clicker still under his hand as an infomercial attempted to get its viewers to purchase gym equipment designed to "Build Abs. She'll Notice—Guaranteed."

She'd finally agreed to discuss Chuck's legal papers, but she didn't have the heart to wake him. Carefully retrieving the remote, she turned off the television. At the bookshelf, she ran her fingers over the spines of her father's classics, her eyes drawn to the "Charlie" journal on the bottom shelf. Charlotte glanced at Chuck and pulled it out. Nestling onto the couch, she burrowed under a blanket and flipped through the pages. Paragraph after paragraph of her father's writing breezed by. Every few pages started with a date and Charlotte's age written in parentheses.

> *Charlotte – (3 hours)*
> *She's a beautiful little thing. She's got my hair—thick and dark and sticking out in all directions, like she's just stuck her finger in an electric socket. Beautiful, tiny Charlotte. She's got a set of lungs on her, too. Screamed bloody loud the moment she popped out of the chute. Hasn't stopped cooing and crying since. She gets that from Elise. Noisy creatures, girls. But the smarter of the sexes. I bet Charlotte has that in spades.*
> *My heart feels so full, but heavy at the same time. She's so tiny, I fear I'll break her. What do I do? How do I protect her? It's a brand-new ballgame. I can't imagine what's in store for my daughter, but I want the world for her. I want the moon and the stars and the lake and the trees. I want her to grow up strong and independent. Intelligent and kind. I want that for my Charlotte. I want all that for my little Charlie.*

The journal fell from Charlotte's limp fingers.

Charlie.

She looked at her father. Chuck lay still, his laugh lines relaxed in slumber.

Her fingertip sought the faint indented lines already branching out from the corners of her own eyes. She'd aged more than she should have in 28 years, the past month and a half having made an indelible mark.

She'd never expected to still be in Lakeside by December. When you didn't want it to, time had a way of going too slow or too fast. For her father, time would eventually stand still. The Alzheimer's would rob him of the ability to form new memories or to hold onto the ones he already had. She re-read the journal entry, imagining Chuck looking down at her, just a few hours old, and seeing himself in a miniature version.

It was a memory he would not hold onto forever.

He would lose it, eventually.

Going, going, gone.

Had her father been prepared for, or even wanted, parenthood? Had Elise talked him into it? He'd been a proud father in the beginning, at least. She stroked the edge of the journal. With a twinge of guilt, she returned it to its rightful place on the bookshelf. For all the times she'd demanded her parents not read her own journal when she was young, she'd never expected to sneak-read her father's decades-old entries.

About her—Chuck's not-so-tiny Charlie.

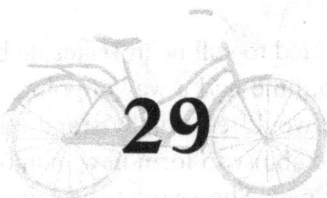

29

Bam.

Charlotte buried her head further under the covers, the disruption to her sleep unidentified. Fuzzy.

Bam.

The second sound, more concrete, prompted her to roll over and seek the usual gray-white dawn over the lake. The morning ritual was something she'd missed while living in Pittsburgh—being greeted by a view of the water from her window before getting out of bed.

But the water wasn't there, that she could see. It was still dark outside.

Charlotte glanced at her phone charging on the bedside table.

3:03 a.m.

A murmur of voices—Adam and Chuck— drifted from downstairs.

And another clang of dishes.

What the hell?

Charlotte threw her legs over the edge of the bed. Her feet hit cold, wooden slats. The lack of insulation between the first floor and second in the old cottage did nothing for toe warmth or sound barrier. She grabbed a pair of socks and jammed her feet into them. Throwing on a zip-up and sweatpants over her pajamas, she strode down the hall. A faint light shone from the first floor, and an acrid scent of something burning stung Charlotte's nostrils. She dashed down the stairs and came to a halt in the doorway of the kitchen.

"Is everything okay?"

Chuck turned from the sink. He was washing a blackened frying pan. "'Mornin', Charlie."

"What's going on?"

Adam looked up from flipping a pancake on a plug-in griddle. Beside it sat a plate mounded with light, golden-brown offerings. Burnt rounds lay in a heap in the trashcan beside the counter.

"Pancakes?" Charlotte met Adam's somewhat desperate gaze. "What's with the pancakes?"

"Dad got up a little early. I heard him making breakfast, so I came down to help."

"It's just after three in the morning."

"He was doing this on the gas stove. I figured the griddle would be safer."

"Oh." *This could have been bad. Very, very bad.* "Have we ever made pancakes in the middle of the night before?"

Adam shook his head. "Not that I know of. So, um, I have to get up in a couple of hours for school. I've got tests tomorrow."

"You mean today." Charlotte plucked the spatula from her brother's hand. "I'll take over, Adam. It's okay. Go get some sleep."

"Thanks, man." Grabbing three pancakes from the stack, Adam turned toward the stairs. "Later."

Charlotte waited until he disappeared.

"Did you realize it was just after three in the morning, Dad?"

The pan in Chuck's hand was clean of residue, but he continued to rub it methodically, his gaze pinned to the surface. He rubbed and rubbed, his hands working separately from his brain.

"Dad?" Charlotte removed the pan from her father's hands and set it on the counter.

Chuck twisted the towel.

Looked at it.

Placed the rolled fabric across the back of his neck, as if he'd just come off the gym floor.

"Your mom used to make you pancakes when you were a kid, Charlie." Chuck tugged on each end of the towel. "You remember?"

"I remember."

"I never made them, but she always liked to. She'd get up early and have them waiting for you when you came down to get on the bus. You loved them. Waffles, too, but not as much. You used to eat at least half a dozen pancakes in a sitting."

"Sure. I still love pancakes."

"I knew you'd like some."

"Sure, Dad."

"Where'd that boy go?"

"What?"

"The boy who was helping me."

"Adam?"

"Adam." Chuck's statement wasn't a question, more like a reminder. "Yes, Adam."

"Your son Adam has school tomorrow."

Chuck's cloud of confusion settled into a semblance of clarity. "Yes. Of course, he does."

Oh, Dad.

Charlotte sighed. "Let's finish up and then we can eat."

"Eat?"

"The pancakes. We'll finish baking them off, then we can eat."

"That sounds lovely."

"Yeah, I think so, too." Charlotte gently pulled the towel from her father's neck and draped it over the sink. While using up the remaining pancake batter, she aimed Chuck toward the cupboard and instructed him to take the plates and silverware to the dining table. Like leading a child, she asked him twice to get the butter and eventually pulled it from the fridge herself.

"Thanks, kid." Chuck frowned at the tub she placed in his hand.

"And here's the syrup." Charlotte fetched it from the pantry. "You can put them both on the table."

It was nearly four o'clock by the time they each sat down to a plateful of pancakes. They ate in silence. Charlotte propped her head on her hand and struggled to stay awake as she processed this newest development. Wide-eyed, Chuck worked away at his food until he'd cleaned his plate of every crumb. He smacked his lips, and Charlotte offered him a napkin.

"That was delicious, Charlie. Thank you for making... pancakes."

"No problem. Your idea, not mine."

Chuck's brows furrowed. Suddenly, he reached across the table, his hand grasping hers with a grip so strong it was sure to leave a mark. Charlotte jumped in her seat but didn't pull away.

"I need to tell you."

"What?"

"I'm sorry." Her father leaned forward. His free hand crept up to his face, holding his cheek as if his head might come apart in pieces. His eyes glistened with tears.

"Oh, Dad. Sorry for what? For the pancakes?"

"I'm sorry, Charlie." Chuck paused. "I'm sorry for not being a better dad. I'm sorry I missed... I missed so much. I'm sorry I wasn't around for your games. I'm sorry for never making pancakes."

"I know." Charlotte looked down at her hand in his.

"I'm getting worse."

"It's okay, Dad."

Chuck wiped his eyes with his napkin.

"I just wanted you to know that. I wanted you to know I'm sorry."

"I know."

"Please stay, Charlie."

Charlotte stared at her empty plate.

"Please."

30

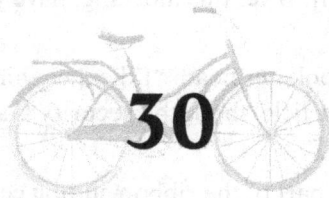

A week later, Charlotte stepped into the hallway leading to *The Lakeside Line*. Though it was just after dawn, the newspaper door was ajar, and light filtered out.

"Merry Christmas Eve, Kate." Charlotte put her coat on the hook, and Kate looked up from her computer, setting jingle bell earrings tinkling. She wore an antler headband and what looked like brown fleece pajamas shoved into suede boots. "Wow. All you need is a red nose."

Kate grinned. "Chuck always likes it when I dress for the holiday, so I wore these to bed last night."

"Very festive," Charlotte said. "Not sure he'll make it in today, though. Hasn't been here much since pancake night. I'll have to take your picture."

"You're up early." Kate returned her attention to the screen. "So, did you get some sleep last night, then?"

"Not exactly. I found a box of albums and trophies in the attic yesterday, and Adam stayed up late looking through baseball photos with Dad. I went to bed early. I got about four hours in before going on Chuck duty. His schedule is so messed up, he didn't fall asleep until almost five o'clock. Seemed pointless for me to go back to bed, so here I am."

"You'll be exhausted by noon."

"Probably, but it was totally worth it. Dad told us some great stories last night. Besides, now it will be easier to get the issue to the printer on time." Charlotte glanced at the notes covering the worktable, honing in on one with Franco Bellimer's name on it. "You haven't seen Mr. B yet this morning, have you? I've got to talk to him."

"Nope." Kate shook her head. "I'd expect him any time, though. He still owes us an article about the security system they're putting in at the high school."

"Dana should be part of the ribbon-cutting ceremony," Charlotte said. "That would be worth a pic, for sure."

"It's impressive she convinced the district to get on board so quickly."

"Agreed." Charlotte walked to the printer, where a fresh stack of papers waited. "This everything?"

"Almost. Give it one last look. You can redline it on the hard-copy."

"Thanks." Charlotte snagged the end-of-year issue and dropped the copies onto her father's work table—*her* work table. The front page featured Charlotte's story about the high school stadium funding and included a picture of Jenny Warren receiving a huge facsimile of a check from Randy Stanner, one of the primary donors for the project.

Taking her father's place, although temporarily, had been an easier transition than Charlotte anticipated, thanks to Kate and Franco guiding her every step of the way.

"Looking forward to a week's break?" Charlotte checked the calendar. "We'll throw together a special edition for the businesses after the first of the year. I want to highlight the new advertisers we added in December."

"How many?" Kate said.

"About a dozen. The community support kind of surprised me."

"Wow. That's great."

The Stanners had helped by talking it up, and each new business owner Charlotte met welcomed her with a smile, a handshake, and, usually, a story about her father. Even if her successes had more to do with Chuck, and all of his connections, than it did with her questionable sales skills, Charlotte was pleased.

Proud, even.

Her low-pressure pitch had translated into a significant increase in advertising dollars.

Charlotte poured herself a mug of coffee and scanned the ads first, confirming every business that had placed one was actually in the layout and had signed off on a final proof. She had begun proofing the news stories by the time Franco Bellimer rolled in.

"Morning." Bellimer dusted snowflakes from his tweed jacket and tossed his leather briefcase into a corner. He dropped down in the chair across from Charlotte. "Looks like we've got ourselves a white Christmas. Supposed to get two to three inches this afternoon, but the temperature isn't dropping too low. How are edits coming? Mostly minor this time?"

"So far." Charlotte laid her pen on the stack of papers. "Everything is pretty clean, now that I'm working on the copy for an hour or two every day."

"Good. You'll get the hang of the timeline. It takes a bit of practice."

"You sticking around for a few minutes, so we can talk?" Charlotte said.

"Of course. Whatever you need."

"Hey, Mr. B." Kate popped her head out of her office door. "I'm still waiting on the latest security piece. Are we doing that this week? I saved you space on page three."

"Sorry." Bellimer shook his head. "They've run into some problems with the wiring. The project is delayed. They'll need a change order or two, which means more money."

"That's too bad," Charlotte said. "Dana will be disappointed."

"They'll figure it out. You know how things go around here—slow as the ferry in a windstorm. I've got something on the animal shelter to fill the hole. Five hundred words okay?"

"Sure." Kate retreated into her office. "But I need it, like, right now."

Bellimer pulled his laptop from his briefcase. "Sending. I'm giving you three pics. Use whatever you want, but definitely the one of the poodle mix. He's named Puddles, and he's been there a month."

Kate laughed, sending her earrings jingling. "They'll never find someone to adopt him with a name like Puddles."

"Ah, come on," Charlotte said. "Poor guy is probably just misunderstood." She handed a page to Franco. "Can you check the last paragraph on your receding shoreline piece, Mr. B? Verb tense right on that? Sounds off."

Bellimer glanced over the copy. "Good catch." He grabbed Charlotte's red pen and made a notation. "You know, you'd be pretty fantastic at this."

Here we go again. Charlotte abruptly got up from her chair to refill her coffee mug. "I'm not staying, Mr. B. I've told you. I'm just here until we can figure something out. That's what I wanted to talk to you about today."

"Oh? How so?" Bellimer leaned back in his chair, threw one of his legs over a knee, and joined his hands on his stomach. His thumbs began tap, tap, tapping.

Charlotte picked up the note with Mr. B's name on it. "Dad and I discussed it. When he steps down as editor, you should take his place."

The little man tilted his head to the side, Charlotte his subject to study. "No, thank you."

"That's it? You won't even consider it? Talk about it?"

"Nope, but I appreciate the offer."

"Why?" Charlotte asked.

"Why do I appreciate the offer, or why won't I consider it?"

"Consider it, of course."

"Because you were made for this."

Charlotte shook her head. "I've told you a million times, Mr. B. I've got a job in Pittsburgh, and I don't want to stay here. I just want to make sure Dad and Adam are okay. I figure I can come up a few days once a month to check on things, meet with advertisers, go to doctor appointments, whatever. We'll probably have to hire a caregiver to stay with Dad, eventually, but I think we can work out something with friends, until things get really bad. I'll do a lot remotely, but someone has to be the face of this paper."

"Yep." Bellimer nodded. "That face should be Chuck Sutton's daughter."

"No, Mr. B."

"Exactly right. 'No' is my answer."

"Don't you want to help?"

"Of course, I do." Bellimer's thumbs thumped away at his stomach. He stared at Charlotte, his eyes small and piercing. She'd seen that look before. She was back in journalism class being graded on her ability to self-edit her own grammatical errors.

You can't make up my mind for me.

"You're just being stubborn, Mr. B."

"Pot. Kettle. Black."

"I've never wanted to be a journalist." Charlotte shook her head. "And editor for my father's newspaper? Even less."

"Just because you never wanted something doesn't mean you don't want it now. Or that it isn't right for you. You're damned good at this. Perhaps better than your dad, even, in his prime."

"I vote with Mr. B on this one," Kate said from her office. "Just so you know."

"Didn't ask," Charlotte said.

"Don't care. He's right."

237

"Stop. Just stop. I don't have time to talk about this right now." Charlotte rubbed her temples—the start of a headache coming on. "I've got to finish my edits."

Bellimer grinned. "You brought it up."

"Fine. Now I'm shutting it down." Charlotte pulled the pile of papers toward her. "Let me finish so we can all enjoy Christmas. We can talk about this again after the new year. Right now, I just need to worry about the final issue."

Bellimer snorted. "Avoidance. That's a gift you've got there, girl." He reached for his coat. "You want me to chew over anything else before I go ask that crazy, old woman to fix me some breakfast?"

"I'm good."

"After, I thought I'd stop in and visit your dad a bit," Bellimer said. "We can watch some sports, if he's up for it."

"Oh, my gosh. Thank you so much. I doubt he or Adam will be out of bed for a couple more hours, though. It was a long night for all of us. Actually, can you ask Bea to fix the boys some breakfast, too, and take it over? She can put it on the newspaper's tab. If no one is up yet, stick it in the fridge."

"No problem." Franco Bellimer threw the strap of his satchel over a shoulder. "You two have a very merry Christmas with your families. I'm going to take one last crack at convincing Bea to join me for a meal tomorrow. She says she's got other plans, but I think she's just being difficult. We should spend Christmas together, rather than both being alone."

"Actually, Bea *does* have plans—she's coming to our place for lasagna," Charlotte said. "And you should, too. Last-minute invite. Six o'clock?"

Bellimer's eyes lit up. "Love to. Thanks."

"You're always welcome, Mr. B. You're practically family."

Bellimer nodded. "Look, I'm sorry I keep pushing the paper. I do want what's best for your dad. I also want what's best for you. Really."

"I know."

"You'll straighten it out. It'll all come together eventually." Franco offered Charlotte a sympathetic smile and opened the door to leave. Bea stood in the open frame.

"Well, hello, Gorgeous." Franco stepped back and gave the marina owner a once-over. "Looking fetching as always this fine morning."

"Out of my way, you old fart."

"Fetching. Simply fetching. I was just coming to ask you to fix me a bite."

Bea waved her hand, dismissing Bellimer. "Keep your drawers on. I'll be back in a minute. Gotta talk to Charlie. Holy Hell. Needy, needy, needy."

"Ah, now, don't get your flannel shirt in a twist, love. I'm not in any hurry. I'll wait as long as it takes... the rest of my life, if necessary." Bellimer motioned Bea forward and gave her a light pat on the lower back.

Bea spun around. "Lecherous old fool."

"Takes one to know one." Franco scooted out the door. "Dinner at Sutton's Choice tomorrow. Guess you're stuck with me, after all."

Charlotte and Kate laughed, and Bea ducked her head back around the door jamb. She'd been letting her buzz cut grow for the cold months, and tufts of downy gray stuck out from her scalp like a newborn gosling.

"Think we're funny, do you?"

"Hell, yes," Kate said. "Half the reason I'm still working here. Very entertaining."

"I suppose there's that." Bea hesitated. "Well, girls, I come to talk to you about the marina."

Charlotte pushed her edits aside and gave the bar owner her full attention. Kate's nails went silent on the keys, and her earrings made nary a *tink*.

"Come on in, Bea." Charlotte motioned to the chair across from her desk. "Is something wrong?"

"Nothin' wrong. Not exactly." Bea shrugged and leaned against the door frame. "I just wanted to ask your intentions. I'm meetin' with Grant Warren soon, see? We're finally talkin' about partnering together. I'm 62. Can't be doin' this forever, but I've put my whole life into it. I've barely got two nickels scraped together for retirement, and, well, my health isn't what it used to be. Got some lumps and bumps I've been gettin' checked out. Business opportunity like this lands in my lap, I gotta take it."

"Oh." *Shit.*

"Looks like you've caught on to the runnin' of the paper right quick, Charlie. I know ya been tryin' to figure things out for Chuck."

"I thought I'd have more time." Charlotte tapped her red pen on the stack of papers in front of her. Despite—or because of—Bellimer's constant pushing, the management of the paper *did* come naturally to her. For the first time in her writing career, she had freedom. She did what she wanted from wherever she wanted to do it. Her writing flowed in Lakeside; she'd written articles for *The Lakeside Line*, of course, but also a personal essay about living with an Alzheimer's patient, something she planned to send to a national magazine. Her split time with the ad agency had also worked out, though she'd promised to return to Pittsburgh no later than March. All the balls she had in the air were still, surprisingly, in the air. It was temporary. Every ball could come tumbling down in a single, fleeting moment.

"I don't mean to pressure ya', Charlie, but the space your dad has been renting needs to be part of the talkin' with Grant. If you don't plan to carry on with the paper, we'll need to think about another renter or if we want to expand the bar. Just tryin' to weigh everything out."

"Of course." Charlotte glanced out the window. A lone seagull, oblivious to the grenade just launched, swooped down and landed on one of the many shrink-wrapped boats waiting out the offseason in the parking lot. "Of course, but even if Dad steps down as editor, he'll want to keep the paper going. He loves it." Charlotte shrugged. "Whether I'm here or not, he'll figure something out."

Bea shrugged. "He'll try his best, but your daddy isn't going to be able to continue much longer by himself. He'll want it done right, or not at all. You know that, much as I do."

"We'll deal with it, even if I have to do more work remotely."

"Had any luck finding an editor?"

"Not exactly," Charlotte said. "I asked Mr. B to take over."

Bea snorted. "Didn't want it, did he?"

"No. He thinks I should stay."

"Huh, well he does know a thing or two. Don't dare tell him I said so, or he'll get an inflated ego. The shit. Grant and me ain't meetin' until the end of the month. How 'bout you ponder it over the holiday and talk with your dad. You can get back to me. That be all right?"

Charlotte nodded. A lump formed in her throat as she pulled forward a block of notes and wrote, in large, red letters, "BEA—JANUARY DEADLINE."

Bea grabbed the doorknob behind her. "It'll be all right. Hell in a handbasket, I know this is a lot to figure, child. I wouldn't want to be in your sneakers."

Bea turned and bolted back down the hall. A muted thump signaled the bar door closing behind her. Silence settled on *The Lakeside Line.*

Kate inched from her office and sat down in the chair across from Charlotte's. "I wouldn't want to be in your sneakers either."

"Hell in a handbasket. What next?"

A muffled chuckle came from Kate, and something in Charlotte broke free. Laughter poured from her uncontrolled, the kind she wasn't sure she could reign in. Her chest hurt from the effort, and, just as quickly, she stopped with a hiccup. A tear snaked down her cheek.

"It'll be all right." Kate handed her a tissue.

"Yeah. Maybe."

Charlotte swiped her face and plucked up the Franco Bellimer note. With shaking fingers, she crumpled the paper into a ball and threw it across the room. It arced just left of the basket and fell to the floor, joining a small pile of crumpled sisters and brothers—a pile Charlotte had added to daily for weeks.

Airball.

My life in a snapshot.

"I'll have to worry about it later." Charlotte pulled the draft of the newspaper forward. "I'll get you the final edits in just a few."

"It'll be all right," Kate repeated.

Charlotte sighed. "Sure."

Within the hour, they had finished and were preparing to leave. Charlotte neatened her desk, and the pink note in the upper right corner of the table caught her eye. She could recite the frayed and faded slip of paper by heart.

She also could no longer ignore it.

Forcing herself across the room, she opened the bottom drawer of the filing cabinet and pulled out the envelope with "CHARLIE" scrawled across it.

31

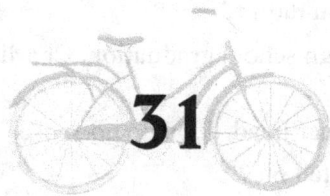

Charlotte sat down across from her father. "Dad, we need to talk."

"What is it, Charlie? What's wrong?"

Charlotte placed the envelope right side up on the kitchen table. "I'd like to go over your legal papers."

Chuck slowly raised his gaze to meet Charlotte's. "Now?"

Charlotte eyed her father, looking for any signs of confusion. Was it a good day or bad?

"Yes, now, if you're up to it. I think it's time." Charlotte opened the flap, hesitated, and tipped the end of the envelope. The contents slid out onto the dining table.

"Oh!"

On top of the small stack of legal papers lay a picture of Charlotte paperclipped to a small card. She picked up the photo. Clearly taken from a distance, it was of her in her college graduation cap and gown. Charlotte pulled the card from behind the photo. It was a graduation invitation.

"Carnegie Mellon?"

She slowly opened it. A note in her father's handwriting graced the upper corner.

I'm so very proud of you, Charlie. You're in the big leagues now, kid. Love, Dad.

"What? I don't understand." Charlotte looked at her father. "Did you... did you *come* to my college graduation?"

Chuck nodded. "I did."

"But I thought you didn't."

"I missed your high school graduation, Charlie. I wasn't about to miss your college."

Charlotte shook her head. It made no sense.

"Why didn't you tell me?"

"I didn't want to make it awkward. It was your special day."

"And Mom wouldn't have been happy?"

Chuck shrugged. "Well, yeah. It was just easier this way. If no one knew I was there."

Oh. My. God.

He'd come. He'd actually come.

"I'm so sorry," Charlotte said. "I thought all this time that... well, I just wish I'd known."

"You know now."

Charlotte placed her hand over her father's and squeezed. "I do. Thank you for coming."

Charlotte didn't know how to proceed. She carefully placed the photo and invitation back into the envelope.

"Do you still want to go over the papers?" Chuck mumbled.

"Are there any more surprises?"

"Yes."

Charlotte sighed and pulled the stack of pages toward her.

* * * * *

Ten minutes later, she took a deep breath and laid the final sheet on the pile.

"I have so many questions."

Chuck's eyes closed. "I expected as much, kid. What do you need to know?"

"I guess I don't understand what you really expect of me. If things get bad—"

"They will," Chuck said. "You know that. We both know that. You heard what the doctor said, same as I did, kid. It's not a matter of 'if,' but 'when.' My health will go south eventually, even with the meds."

"Fine," Charlotte said. "When things get bad, what exactly do you want of me?"

Chuck took her hand. "I want you to run the paper—keep it alive for the community—and I want you to claim what is yours, of course." His hand swept the air, encompassing the kitchen and all that surrounded them. "Sutton's Choice."

"What?"

Chuck nodded. "The house has been in my family for generations, and *you're* my family. That's why your mother and I agreed it would not be part of the divorce settlement. It's in a trust, along with a fair amount of assets. I've been pretty smart with my investments over the years, and when I die—"

"I don't understand."

"Sutton's Choice is yours, Charlie. I've listed you as the successor trustee and beneficiary. I've just been keeping it up for you, hoping someday you'd want to come back to home base."

"But what about Adam?"

"He would live here, too, until he's 18, and then it's up to you. Either way, he gets his own financial share when he turns 23. College first, though. He has a college fund. You're both taken care of. I've set everything up."

"But Sutton's Choice is your home."

"Probably not much longer." Chuck let out a breath, as if he'd been holding it for a very long time. "I've made plans to go to the memory care unit where my mother was when my health gets too bad. There's an account for that, too, of course."

Charlotte frowned. "You've got plenty of time, Dad."

"You don't know that." Chuck shook his head. "Neither of us knows that. That's why I've got everything ready to go. The financial and healthcare power of attorney papers, the trust, a living will." Chuck motioned to the envelope between them. "And my last will and testament, of course. Did everything long ago, before my memory really began to strike out. I have you listed as my POA for everything. If you refuse, Franco is my back-up, but then there's the matter of legal guardianship."

"Legal guardianship? Of Adam?" Charlotte said.

"Franco thinks he's too old to raise him. I considered asking Jake, but really, it should be family. I'd prefer it be you. At 14, Adam has a say in the matter, but I'd feel better knowing you were willing."

Leaning back, Charlotte stared at her father. Her fingers sought the flap of the envelope in front of her, rolling it and folding it and rolling it again. The anxiety she had tried to tamp down for months threatened, again, to suffocate her.

"So, you essentially want me to keep the newspaper alive, take over a 100-year-old house, handle your finances, and raise a 14-year-old brother I didn't know I had."

"Yeah, kid. That pretty much sums it up."

"Adam barely tolerates me, Dad."

"You're exaggerating." Chuck tugged his hair, sending the messy, dark strands into further disarray. "He's a teenager, and I didn't promise it would be roses. I think he'll come around to the idea of you being his guardian, though, if it comes to that. I know it's a lot."

"That's an understatement." Charlotte turned the envelope over, her name face-down. "How can you possibly think I'd be the best person to take care of him?" Charlotte waved her hand just as her father had done. "And all of this?"

"Because this place is meant for you. You belong here. You're what Adam needs, and maybe he's what you'll need, as I get worse.

Look, this isn't just about the practical or material things, Charlie. This isn't just about a house or a job. It's about our family. I spent so much time on the road while you were growing up—so much time living out of a suitcase and missing out on birthday parties and games and such. I've come home. I'll die here, among my friends—in a place I love, doing something I love, with people I love. I wish I could turn back time, so I could do a few things over, but I can't. You're my family. What I really want is for you to be happy. That's what I've always wanted."

"I understand, but—"

"You can find that here, Charlie. Lakeside is like no other place. You belong here, and so does Adam. It's your choice."

"That's a hell of a choice." Charlotte's heart raced with confusion and an old, familiar resentment. Who the hell was he to tell her where she belonged?

"Your choice to make," Chuck said.

No choice.

* * * * *

By early Christmas morning, Franco Bellimer's predicted snowfall lay like a thick blanket on the waterfront lawn. Ice crystals weighed heavy on the trees, bending the limbs low to the ground. There was a quiet about the small community, as if everyone had hunkered down and would hibernate until spring.

While Chuck took a proper rest in his room before everyone converged on the house for Christmas dinner, Charlotte sat on the couch with her father's journal open in her lap. On a branch just outside the living room window, a cardinal contrasted against the white backdrop. It was unusual to see so much snow this early in the winter, turning Sutton's Choice into a cozy cocoon.

Charlotte returned her attention to the journal in her hands. The few entries she'd read had provided a gift—an insight she'd craved nearly all her life.

She'd discovered, in some small part, how her father felt about being a dad.

How he parented. How he loved.

For her, the journal was the most meaningful thing her father had ever written. Much like Charlotte with her own journal, Chuck had poured everything he was feeling—all his dreams and insecurities as a person and a parent—onto the pages in indelible ink.

> *Charlie: age 3*
>
> *I traveled a lot this month. Came in on a red-eye last night from Boston, so I could take my little girl to a Toledo Mud Hens game today. Before Charlie, I barely looked back when I got on a plane. Now, I feel pulled in two directions. I'm starting to realize I barely know my daughter. She's a mystery to me... one I'm not sure I'll ever have enough time to solve. Elise handles everything. I'd like to say I feel bad about that, but not really. Purple dresses with satin ribbons, dolls with half their clothes missing, stuffed teddy bears. Hell, I don't know how to interact with any of it. I always thought I'd have a boy. Boys aren't mysterious, but Charlie sure is.*
>
> *Today I got us seats right behind the dugout down the first base line. I bought cotton candy and thought we were having a grand old time. In the third, a fly ball came right at us. I caught it and handed it to Charlie. She looked at it, looked at me, looked at it again, then chucked the thing back out onto the field. She looked so proud of herself, her bright eyes and freckles framed by that dark hair beneath the baseball cap I'd bought her.*
>
> *"Ball, Daddy." She pointed at the pitcher. "Baseball?" I shook my head, sorry to tell her it was no longer ours. Charlie looked up at me with those big eyes, then back at the pitcher. Then she cried—not just a whimper but howling gasps. We left early, and I couldn't console her all the way home. When we got back to the house, I snagged an old ball from a box of memorabilia and handed it to Charlie. She stopped crying immediately and smiled up at me, offering the ball right back. "Baseball, Daddy?" She seemed more pleased to give it to me than she'd seemed receiving it.*

Girls. I'll never understand them.

Charlotte didn't remember the game, but she could read between the lines. Since she *could* remember, Chuck had loved baseball. He'd breathed it, ate it, slept it. Charlotte assumed, even at three, she'd wanted to make him proud and "play ball." She'd thrown the ball onto the field to show him she could do it, and then she'd offered him the second baseball as a gift from daughter to father.

Where's the mystery in that?

Stretching, she placed the journal back on the shelf and walked into the kitchen. Adam sat writing in a notebook. His Language Arts book lay open on the table.

"They're still giving kids homework over the holiday break, huh? What's your project?"

"It's stupid," Adam said. "An essay about what I want most in the new year."

"Would you like some help?"

"Meh." He shrugged and twisted a piece of dark hair that had breached the edge of his hoodie. "I'm not Dad, if that's what you're thinking."

"I'm not. And just for the record, I'm not Dad either. Nowhere close." Charlotte pulled a chair over. "Can I take a look?"

Again, the shrug. "You won't like it."

"You don't know that."

Should she be amused or annoyed? She recognized her own teen-angsty self in Chuck's son. Pulling Adam's story across the table, Charlotte stifled the urge to pick up his pencil and start editing. Instead, she leaned back in her seat and got comfortable.

> *What I Want Most*
> *by Adam Sutton*
> *My dad, Chuck Sutton, wasn't always in my life. He didn't know he had a son until my mom dropped me off five years ago. Chuck took me in, even though I was a stranger.*

He's given me the best years of my life, but in the past several months, Dad has been drifting away, kind of like a piece of wood swept out into the middle of the lake.

The doctor thinks Dad has Alzheimer's Disease. What I want most is to spend as much time as I can building memories with him. Five years could never be enough. I feel like I've only just started to know who he is, just as he is becoming someone else. It isn't fair to him, and it isn't fair to me. I guess the memories my dad and I make now will be for me more than him.

For Chuck Sutton, those memories will eventually float away, out to the middle of the lake like that piece of wood, and be no more.

Charlotte jumped up from the table. Swallowing back tears, she rushed to the sink and faced the window.

The guilt.

Charlotte had 18 years with Chuck. She didn't remember exactly when she started to hate him for being a shitty father, but she was pretty sure she'd gotten more than five good years out of the relationship.

"You're a very good writer, Adam."

A mumbled "thanks."

"When you think you're done, I'm happy to proofread it, just to make sure you don't have any grammatical issues," Charlotte said. "If you'd like."

A mumbled "sure."

Chuck had taught her to sail. On very rare occasions, he had played dress-up with her—badly. He'd painted her nails and conjured stories starring Yogi Bear-a and the rest of her stuffed animal collection. He had bought her the dollhouse with its miniature Sutton family who moved from room to room to room.

He'd tried being a father.

And then he hadn't.

His success with *Smokin' Smokey Joe* had taken that away. Taken *him* away. Her father had even removed himself from his family, had chosen to *stay* away for the good of the family, because he and Elise were no longer getting along. He'd made that choice.

But when it came to Adam, neither father nor son had had a choice. Chuck hadn't known Adam existed for the first nine years of his son's life.

In Charlotte's case, she'd walked away from Lakeside and never looked back. She'd chosen to deny Chuck time with her for ten long years.

And denied herself, as well.

Her father had chosen to let her.

They were both at fault for the relational divide they'd created in the past decade. She could have reached out just as easily as he could have.

So many choices. So much hurt.

Charlotte washed her hands at the sink, dabbed a dish towel to her eyes, filled a glass with water, and gulped it down. She filled another.

Finally, she turned. Adam glanced up from his essay.

"I'm going for a quick ride around the peninsula." Charlotte grabbed her coat and put on her boots. "The lasagna is in the refrigerator. I'll be back in time to heat it up for dinner. Jake's bringing Sydney over, and Bea and Franco are coming."

"Cool."

Charlotte reached for the door knob.

"Yeah," Adam said, "so if you could look at my essay later, when I'm done... um, that would be okay, I guess."

Charlotte looked over her shoulder and smiled. "No problem."

It would be a good one. How she'd make it through the final edits, she had no idea.

32

PRESCHOOL

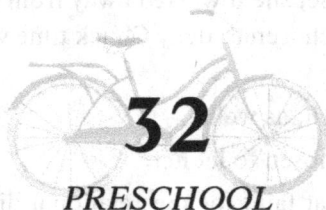

Four-year-old Charlotte could barely keep her eyes open.

But she must. How else could she catch Santa in the act?

She rolled over in her twin bed. Facing the door, she snuggled Yogi Bear-a against her cheek, lowering her eyelids to a slit so she could still see through her lashes. Santa would never guess she was awake. She'd make sure to snore.

Pony. Pony. I hope he brings a pony.

But she'd like a puppy, too, which would take up less space in her bedroom. Or maybe it would be the dollhouse Daddy had shown her in the city. A dollhouse would be nice, her own Sutton's Choice with a mommy and a daddy and a sister and a brother.

Charlotte strained to hear the big guy in red and his sleigh with eight tiny reindeer. Would they land on the roof just a few feet above her? How did Santa get in? The cottage didn't have a fireplace, but she always got Christmas presents.

He must get in somehow.

Charlotte rubbed her feet together. The footed pajamas Mommy had made her wear to bed so she'd be in something red and green and cute for pictures on Christmas morning itched something

252

terrible. Suddenly, the second stair from the top—the one that needed fixing—creaked.

She always hopped over it.

Santa wouldn't know that.

Charlotte's heart hammered so loud she was sure he would hear. The whole house would hear. And if she scared Santa away, there'd be no presents.

No pony. No puppy. No dollhouse.

She slowed her breaths and began counting to 10, something Daddy had taught her. In. Out. In. Out. Charlotte sunk into the covers and wrapped her arms tighter around Yogi Bear-a. Her eyelids fluttered, and she caught a glimpse of a shadow in the doorway.

She dreamed of the big guy in red and a family and a puppy in a cottage of her own.

33

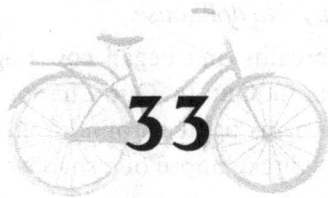

Charlotte failed to return, even briefly, to Pittsburgh. The busy days stretched into weeks and into months, bleeding the old year into the new, then January into February. Though ice fishermen enjoyed a fruitful freeze, The Surly Sturgeon served fewer customers than in winters past. Charlotte, Bea, Franco, Jake, and Chuck, on his good days, played darts and kept the lights on for the handful of regulars who loved the offseason routine of Meatball Mondays, Wednesday Wings, and Thirsty Thursday pitcher night specials.

* * * * *

As if knowing change was, inevitably, just around the corner, the first of March blew in like a lion riding an unexpected Northeaster. Charlotte's boots sunk into the ice with a crunch. The snow covered the waterfront like icing on a wedding cake, the surface so smooth she hated to disturb it on the way to the marina. Though the storm hadn't put down much of the fluffy stuff, a mix of freezing rain dripped like frozen tentacles from the tree limbs and power lines overhead.

She plodded through the parking lot, still a landing zone for boats yet to be put back in the water. Though it was just a few weeks before St. Patrick's Day—the unofficial spring opening for many of the seasonal shops—the surface of the lake still lay frozen in spots. She had forgotten just how beautifully desolate her little patch of Lake Erie could be during the cold months. The lack of people equaled peace, in her mind, and she loved it.

She would miss it.

Looking over her shoulder at Sutton's Choice, Charlotte debated if her dad would get up before noon. The March holiday issue, devoted to St. Patrick's Day, would fall to Charlotte. Her father's nocturnal habits continued to flip-flop. He got up at odd times and often greeted the sunrise long before it was ready to be greeted. The night before, Charlotte had spent the wee hours watching old sitcoms with him.

Friends checked in on him daily, while Charlotte was at the office and Adam at school. It had become a group effort to keep an eye on Chuck, run the newspaper, and deal with Adam's schoolwork and sports activities.

And maintain Charlotte's sanity.

Anywhere else, it might have been different.

Lakeside people did for each other whatever needed done. No grumbling. No excuses. Charlotte shook her head. She was grateful to Bea and Grant for giving her an extension on deciding the fate of the newspaper's rental space. They'd been so patient.

Until today.

She wasn't looking forward to her meeting with them.

Charlotte entered the empty office. Removing her coat, she dropped the envelope containing Chuck's legal documents onto the table, turned on the coffeemaker, and sank down into her father's old leather chair. She wouldn't be alone for long.

With a sigh, she pulled out her phone and re-read her boss' email message.

> *Charlotte,*
> *It's been a pleasure working with you remotely these*

past several months. Despite your father's health issues, you've proven to be reliable, talented, and very professional. We've set up an initial March 15 appointment with our new client, Designer Greens. The build-your-own-salad franchise should be a perfect fit for your skills. With that, we'd like to formally offer you a full-time position with our ad agency. Please call me at your convenience to discuss salary and benefits. Someone with your skills is hard to find, and we hope you'll be a member of the Beyond Business family for many years to come.

— Tania

A noise emanated from the hall, and Grant poked his head in the doorway.

"Good morning," he said. "We're ready for you in the bar."

"Thanks. I'll be right there."

Grant nodded and retreated.

Taking a deep breath, Charlotte pulled the pink note from the corner of the table and read it for the last time—"CHARLIE (daughter), legal papers, bottom file drawer." Slowly, she crumpled the note into a ball. With an overhand flick, it struck the rim of the basketball hoop on the other side of the room and, to her surprise, fell into the trash can beneath.

"Two points," she whispered. "About damned time."

It had taken months, but she'd finally gotten the hang of running the office, just as it no longer mattered. Standing, she crossed to her father's filing cabinet, opened the bottom drawer, and placed the envelope back into its metal coffin.

* * * * *

Charlotte plunked her notepad down on The Surly Sturgeon's bar and set her coffee mug beside it.

"All right." She eyed the full shot glass on the counter in front of her. "What's this?"

"For courage." Bea grinned and held up a glass of her own. She tipped her head back, and the amber liquid disappeared in a flash.

Charlotte grimaced. "Nine in the morning, Bea. It's way too early for courage." Laughing, she pushed the liquor across. "Have at it."

"Suit yourself, girlie." The second drink disappeared as quickly as the first. "What's your pleasure, Grant?"

"I'm good." Grant slid onto a stool. "Jenny fed me one of her protein shakes this morning, and my intestines are still trying to decide if they're happy about it."

"Protein shake?" Bea swiped her hand across her mouth. "Well, shit fire. Bathroom's in the far corner."

The outer door banged open, and a gust of wind preceded a tall woman in a heavy parka. Her white hair sat like a tight cloud of curls against her dark skin.

"Have I come to the right place?" She waved in their direction. "Looks like I did. Good morning, Grant."

"So glad you could make it." Grant motioned to a nearby stool. "Have a seat. Zara Taylor, this is Bea Douglas. She owns the bar. And this is Charlotte Sutton. Her father is the editor of *The Lakeside Line*—the paper I told you about."

"Very nice to meet you."

"Same," Bea said. "Whiskey? Beer? Coffee?"

"No, thank you."

Charlotte nodded a greeting and sized up the stranger. Who was she? Why was she here?

"We invited Zara to sit in on this meeting," Grant said. "We think she might be of help. First, we'd like to hear what your thoughts are, Charlotte, on the matter of the newspaper."

"What's your plan, girl? Plain and simple," Bea said.

Charlotte took a long sip from her coffee mug. She placed it on the counter and spread her hands flat on either side of it.

She couldn't stall any longer.

"First, I just want you to know how much I appreciate you giving me time to come to a decision. I... it's been a struggle."

"Depends on what you mean by that, Charlie," Bea said. "I'm

257

not one for compliments, but I think you've done a fine job with the paper."

Grant nodded. "She's right."

"Thank you, but I guess I should just get to the point. I've been offered a full-time job with the ad agency in Pittsburgh."

"And you want to take it?" Bea said.

"I do."

"We expected that, actually," Grant said, "which is why Zara is here." He motioned to the newcomer. "Would you like to explain?"

Zara nodded and pulled a couple of newspapers from the bag she'd hung from her chair. She pushed the stack across the bar to Charlotte. The top paper was the last issue of *The Lakeside Line*.

"What—"

"I'm an editor, and I just moved here from Cleveland." Zara pulled the second newspaper to the top of the pile. "You see, I'm retired, but I'd be willing to help your dad for a year or two. With your support, of course. Running a small community paper could be a very nice change of pace."

"Wait, what?" Charlotte glanced at the newspaper on the bar and back at Zara. "You were an editor for the *Cleveland Teller*?"

"Yes." Zara unfolded the copy of the newly defunct periodical which had provided the news to the entire east side of Ohio for decades. "I was with them for more than 40 years."

"What the heck? How did you hear about *The Lakeside Line*?" Charlotte wiped her sweaty palms on her jeans. "I'd given up on finding someone. Dad was willing to retire, and that's what I was going to tell you all today. Neither of us is happy about it, but it seemed the only way."

"Zara is here at my request," Grant said. "I dabbled in investing with her paper, but they've really struggled in recent years. Obviously. Now they're shuttered."

"It's a loss," Zara said, "but I've always had a vacation home here, so making the move full-time was an easy change. I'll miss my work, though. I'd love to help keep a community paper going, if you and your dad are interested. I might even consider buying it someday, if you decide to sell. This would give me a chance to see if I'd like to own it, eventually."

"Chuck has worked so hard," Grant said. "I don't want to see the paper fail like so many others. I'm willing to invest in both the marina and *The Lakeside Line*, if that works for you, Charlotte. You'll have whatever you need to keep it up, until your family is really ready to make a change. Zara's salary included."

"So, there's really no reason to worry anymore, child," Bea said. "We've got you covered."

Charlotte's breath left her. Would Zara run the paper like her father? What would Chuck think if someone from outside took it over?

"Wow. I don't know what to say."

34

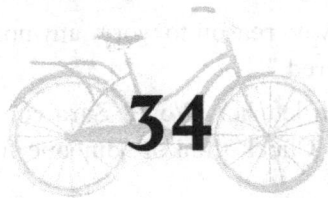

After the early morning meeting, Charlotte returned to the cottage, grabbed her purse and keys, and quickly left out the back door. She sat in her car, her breath fogging the window, and noodled over what had just transpired.

Nothing had gone as she'd expected.

Or *they'd* expected, actually.

What had she done?

With a sigh, she puttered off through town. She slowed to a crawl and exited through the open east gate entrance. To her left was the lake and a natural shoreline ice sculpture, added to with each wave that had fanned up and over the rocks. Winding her way onto the main road of Marblehead, Charlotte pulled into a parking spot in front of The Clip Joint. As was her habit, she leapt over the mat and rammed her shoulder into the door. She turned the knob, practically falling into the shop. The tinkle of bells rang above the buzz of a hairdryer.

"Seriously, girl, you're gonna hurt someone doing that trick." Sammy turned off the gadget but didn't bother to look up from his customer, who happened to be Mrs. T. "I don't think my liability insurance covers homicidal clients."

"Good morning to you, too," Charlotte said. "Hi, Mrs. T. Looking good."

"Hello, dear. Happy early St. Paddy's Day. Cold enough out there for you? I had to pull out the winter gear again for Snuggles." Beaming, Mrs. T held up her Chihuahua. Almost lost in a voluminous kelly-green-and-black-sequined plaid vest and bow tie, the dog's bulbous eyes drilled into Charlotte's with disturbing intent.

Sammy gave an eyeroll over the woman's head.

"Cute," Charlotte said. "I hope it warms up before season starts. This is ridiculous. Sammy, if you have time, I need to talk to you about something."

"In a hurry?"

"No. Dad's asleep on the couch."

"'Kay, I'm almost done here. Mama's in the back, and there's a plate of Christmas cookies if you're interested."

"Geez, how many did she make? It's March."

"I don't know." Sammy shrugged. "Who cares? They freeze, don't they? We'll still be pulling them out for Christmas in July. I'm pretty sure Mrs. T would eat some, wouldn't you?"

Mrs. T's brows rose. "Never met a cookie I didn't like, dear."

"Exactly."

Charlotte walked down the now familiar hall to where Mama Macon was folding laundry.

"Charlotte, sweet girl." The little woman dropped her towel on the table and went in for a hug. "When are you and my boy going to give me grandbabies?"

"Not today, Mama. Not today. Cookies?"

"Above the fridge."

Charlotte fetched the platter featuring Mama's shortbread, chocolate oatmeal cookies, and pecan cups.

"We still have about eight dozen in the freezer," Mama said.

Charlotte stuffed a shortbread in one cheek. Mama's cookies alone could be enough reason to put down roots.

But not a good enough reason.

Charlotte took the tray out to the main cutting area, where Sammy was ringing up Mrs. T at the reception desk.

"Cookie, Mrs. T?"

"Well, of course, dear. Why do you think I'm still here?" Mrs. T's bejeweled hand snapped up three shortbreads and handed one to Snuggles. "Stay warm, darlings." She threw an air kiss, pulled her jacket on over her velveteen jogging suit, and helped Snuggles wave his paw before exiting and sending the bells chiming, yet again. Sammy waited until the door shut and flopped down in his cutting chair.

"What's up, Char? We're shutting down early today. I've got about 20 minutes before my last appointment. It's Rev. Salamon, so get all your bitchin' out now."

"You think that's the only reason I come in here?" Charlotte said. "To bitch about something?"

"Sure. Don't you know your hairdresser is the next best thing to a therapist? Do you need me to cut your hair while you vent? I really should trim up those bangs."

"I like my bangs."

"Suit yourself."

Charlotte pulled the reception chair over and sat down facing Sammy. "Why did you stay here?"

Sammy cocked his head. "What kind of weird-ass question is that?"

"Why did you stay here, instead of going back to Miami or New York or Cleveland or any other big city? You could have owned several salons, by now. You could have been doing haircuts for the stars or your favorite football team, for that matter. Why did you stay here? It's not as if your family was from here."

Sammy sat back. His foot dipped to the floor and sent the chair spinning. He let it go one, two, three rotations and stopped it, precisely, with his toe.

"I like it here. It took a while, but I think *here* likes *me*."

The simple statement punched Charlotte in the gut.

She shook her head. "But we hated high school, Sammy. It was miserable. All we wanted was to get out and as far away as possible."

"Did we?"

"I did. *I* wanted more." Charlotte motioned, encompassing the room. "A hell of a lot more than this."

Sammy's brow arched. "You dissin' The Clip Joint? Get the hell out."

There was a pause.

"Oh, God. I'm so sorry, Sammy. I didn't mean it like it came out. I didn't mean your shop. *Really.* I love your shop."

Sammy burst out laughing. "I know. I'm just messin' with you."

"Ass."

Dipping his toe again, Sammy sent the chair spinning and stopped it squarely in front of Charlotte. "I hated high school, but I also really didn't mind it so much. I mean, it sucked, don't get me wrong, but I had you. We had a lot of fun together."

"True."

"That's what made it all right," Sammy said. "We got through it together. I didn't really care if anyone else liked me."

"What? Are you saying I did?"

"Maybe. Probably. We were kids. Of course, you cared about being liked... about being popular."

"I suppose."

"High school was such a long time ago. By the time I was ready to leave, I realized maybe I didn't want to." Sammy shrugged. "And Mama is here." His gaze strayed from Charlotte's. "Honestly? I hoped you'd eventually come back, too, someday. And now here you are."

"I came back because of Dad's health."

Sammy tilted his head. "Right."

"It's the only reason I've stayed," Charlotte said.

"If you say so. Anyway, I'm pretty sure New York would have been too much for me, Char. I'd rather be the big walleye in the little lake than some tiny shark bait in the ocean."

"That's not quite how that phrase goes."

"Whatever."

"I like the city," Charlotte said. "I don't plan to be shark bait. I'd rather be a shark, someday."

"There's nothing wrong with that. Someone has to be the shark. Heck, around here, you probably already are. None of it matters. Only what *you* want matters. Some people are happy in the city, some aren't. Do you want to stay, or don't you?"

A million bees buzzed in Charlotte's head, trying to escape. "I don't know."

"Bullshit," Sammy said. "You've had months."

Charlotte gave him a look.

Yes, she was stalling. Her prerogative.

"Anyway." Sammy cocked his head, studying her. "Be real with me, Char. Shark or no shark, what do you get in Pittsburgh that you can't get here?"

Charlotte debated. "I can see a show. I can walk wherever I want for a coffee or dinner or whatever."

"How many shows did you go see in Pittsburgh in 10 years?"

"One."

"So, you and I can go see a show in Cleveland or Toledo, instead," Sammy said. "Granted, we can't walk there, but what's an hour drive once every decade? Hell, by the time we'd get around to actually planning such a trip, they might get the stage rights up at the high school. Nearly as good. We can order watery beer and a platter of nachos supreme at The Surly Sturgeon after."

"Smartass."

"Sarcasm. It's my gift, Char." Sammy set his chair spinning. "Just trying to convince you to stay."

She had to tell him.

"The ad agency just made me an offer for a full-time position, Sammy," Charlotte said. "They want me as soon as possible."

Sammy put his foot down, stopping the chair facing away from her.

"I'd be stupid not to take it. It's a significant step up."

Sammy slowly turned the cutting chair around. He didn't hide the familiar sadness in his eyes. "Wow. Good for you, Char."

"Thanks."

"Editor of *The Lakeside Line* would be a step up, too, you know," Sammy said. "That would look great on your resume, even if you just did it for a year or two."

"I need to take this job. There are too many reasons to accept it."

Sammy clasped Charlotte's hands between his own. "I get it. I get it, but there are lots of reasons not to. I want you to stay. Jake wants you to stay."

Another wrinkle in her plans.

"Even Adam wants you to stay," Sammy said. "And for damned sure, your dad does. *Everybody* wants you to stay. These are all great reasons."

Charlotte shook her head. "I should go."

"Should you?" Sammy placed a palm on Charlotte's cheek. "What if... what if we married? I'll even offer to climb The Tree, so Mama can finally get her grandbabies."

"Oh, dear God."

"Or we could have you artificially inseminated with my man swimmers. We'd make beautiful Chammies." Sammy dropped from his chair and leaned on one knee. "Will you—"

Charlotte's eyes widened. "Please tell me you're not serious."

"I could be, if it keeps you here." He rolled her left hand over.

"Get up, Sammy."

"Come on, Char, think about it." Sammy sighed. "You should stay. You're awesome at the paper. Don't you love anything about this place?"

"I love *you*. You're the bomb, Sammy from Miami." Charlotte swallowed. "And you're my best friend."

"'I love you, too, Char. That's what home is—where you are loved."

Charlotte frowned. "Home can be anywhere."

"Can it? Why don't we—"

"I can't marry you, Sammy."

Sammy chuckled, dropped her hand, and pulled himself off the floor. "Yeah. I didn't think you would. I just wanted you to know you've got options." He shrugged and flopped back in his chair.

"Don't scare me like that."

"Offer stands. If Jake doesn't put a ring on it, we could be the most talked-about couple in town."

Charlotte rolled her eyes. "Just what I've always dreamed of."

"I've got your back." Sammy arched a brow. "We've *all* got your back. What about finding an editor for the paper? I didn't think you had any takers."

Charlotte sunk deeper into her chair. "Good news. Bea and Grant figured something out." She explained the morning meeting.

"Shit, Char. That's... great."

"Yeah. I'm a little concerned about letting a stranger run the paper, but—"

"There ya go," Sammy said, slapping the arm of his chair. "Obviously, you should stay."

Charlotte shook her head. "But Zara seems like a great fit. Dad and I can—"

"Dammit, Char." Sammy squinted at her. "You've already made up your mind, haven't you? It's done. You've already made your choice."

Charlotte swallowed. Her voice came out in a squeak.

"I'm sorry."

"You've accepted the Pittsburgh job?"

"Yes, but I'll come back and visit this time," Charlotte said. "A lot. I promise. I'll be back as often as I need to be. Every weekend, if necessary. Dad has already talked to someone about long-term care, and we've got an in-home caregiver scheduled to help him for a few hours every day. I'll be Dad's Power of Attorney."

"What about Adam?"

"Franco and Jake will keep an eye on him, while I'm in Pittsburgh. We've worked it out."

"Oh, Char."

"It'll be okay." Charlotte shrugged, staring down at the black and white checked tile.

"You're really leaving, aren't you?"

"Yes."

"Again?"

Charlotte nodded, barely able to speak. "Yes."

"Dammit," Sammy said. "Well, congratulations, I guess. Shit. I'm proud of you. I'm not happy, but I'm proud of you."

He leaned forward in his chair and his arms snaked around her shoulders. His forehead pressed against hers, and they sat there, knee-to-knee, unmoving. For the briefest of moments, Charlotte kept her emotions in check, but a sob forced its way to the surface. Sammy pulled her tighter, and she buried her face in his shoulder until she'd soaked his t-shirt.

* * * * *

Charlotte hopped over The Clip Joint welcome mat without killing herself. Scrubbing the tears from her cheeks, she got into her car, did a U-turn in the middle of the deserted street, and turned toward Sutton's Choice. She pulled into the hotel parking lot and cut the engine. Her breath plumed white as the car cooled.

She wasn't ready to tell her father and Adam.

Circling the house, she made her way down onto the waterfront path. Footprints of some prior walker and his or her dog preceded Charlotte's trip along the edge of the lake to the snow-covered steps leading to the top deck of the pavilion. The cement dock shone, the area near the flagpole at the end a dangerous, slick sheet of black ice. The lake itself presented a bleak picture, gunmetal gray with patches of snow reaching all the way to Kelleys Island. Since she was little, Charlotte had wanted to walk across the frozen lake but had never had the nerve or stupidity to try. Many years before, a Bay Area student had made the trip on a dare. He'd fallen through a thin patch and died.

The clouds briefly parted, and the lake winked with flashes of sun. She sighed. There was nothing left to think about. She'd take the next two weeks to finalize everything before going back to her new job.

She should be excited. It wasn't like she'd be leaving Lakeside for another decade, and her father could keep the paper. She'd come at Easter or for a long weekend. Or several long weekends. And, again, over Memorial Day and sometime in the summer. She could come anytime she wanted to.

She could have both—a city life and a lakefront getaway.

So why did the prospect of finally getting what she wanted leave her feeling so lost?

Charlotte turned to leave and caught a glimpse of movement near the cottage. Wearing no coat, Adam stood on the front lawn. He yelled something, but the words were lost on the wind.

"Oh, no." Bolting down the pavilion steps, she hurried up the path and stopped just within hearing distance.

"Dad," Adam said. "Where are you?"

Charlotte closed the gap in seconds.

"What's wrong? What happened?"

Adam stood shivering with his arms wrapped around his chest. He shook his head.

"It's Dad. I don't know where he is."

35

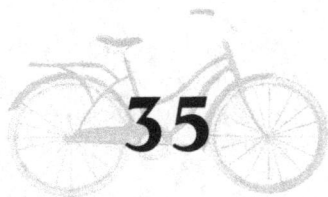

Charlotte pushed her brother into the house.

"Start at the beginning. How long has he been gone?"

"I don't know. I've been up for about an hour. He wasn't watching TV, so I thought he was still asleep. When I checked on him a few minutes ago, he wasn't in his room."

"Shit." Charlotte bounded up the stairs to the second floor.

Panic surged through her.

How could he just disappear?

Each of the upstairs rooms proved empty.

Charlotte returned to the first floor. "He's not here."

"I told you."

Jake burst through the back door.

"I got your message, Adam."

"Oh, thank God," Charlotte said.

Jake threw her a sympathetic look. "It's okay. We'll figure it out."

"But Dad's been gone at least an hour," Adam said. "What do we do?"

"Go put warmer clothes on for starters, while I talk to Charlotte. We'll figure out a plan."

"Right." Adam rushed upstairs.

"I'm so sorry." Jake guided Charlotte to a seat at the table. "Kate is at the bank. She's going to look for him on the main roads on her way back. I already checked, and neither Bea nor Franco has seen him. Any idea where he could have gone? He's not at the marina."

Charlotte shook her head. "He could be anywhere."

She stood and looked out the kitchen window. Her father's SUV sat in the parking lot, covered in snow and ice. The temperatures were expected to fall again by nightfall. If he was on foot, they'd need to find him, and quickly. A tremor ran up her arms, and she braced herself against the kitchen counter with her back to Jake.

"We need to check the perimeter. Walking was always his favorite exercise. He'd do two laps of the fence line every morning."

"Okay," Jake said. "The perimeter. That makes sense."

"I'll do it." Charlotte returned to the table.

Jake pushed a notepad toward her. On it, he had sketched a map of the area. He pointed to the main road through town.

"I'll check the shops," he said. "I doubt much is open, and I can catch up to you if I don't find him first."

"Everything looked closed when I came from The Clip Joint," Charlotte said.

"Your dad wouldn't know that, though... not in his state." Jake touched Charlotte's hand lying, lifeless, on the table. "Maybe I'll bump into Lakeside Security. If not, I'll tell the administration office. They can send someone out."

Adam hurried into the room and pulled his jacket from a hook by the door. "Where do you want me to look?"

"Check the houses on the other side of the marina, please." Jake tapped the map. "Maybe he went to the bar and got confused or made a wrong turn."

"Maybe," Adam said.

The emotions of the morning were too much. Charlotte was on the brink of completely losing control, but control was exactly what she needed. There was fear in her brother's eyes. She could not show her own. Not in that moment.

"Hey. It'll be okay." She rose and tentatively put her arm around Adam's shoulder. He stiffened, but she did not let go. "We'll find him. Dad won't have gone far."

"Sure." Adam pulled away.

Charlotte's shoulders slumped. "You have your cell? Be careful, Adam. The roads are icy."

"Yeah, man. I got it."

"You should walk," Charlotte said. "Don't ride the bike in this mess."

"I *got* it." Adam rushed out the door, allowing it to slam behind him.

Charlotte sighed. "I blew that."

"You didn't. He'll be fine," Jake said.

"I doubt it." Charlotte rifled through a basket by the back door, pulling out gloves and an old beanie cap. "Where the hell could he have gone? Dammit, don't they own anything warmer than this?" She looked down at her shaking hands. The tremors from before moved up her arms, taking over her body.

"It's okay," Jake said.

Charlotte looked at Jake through a haze of tears. "Someone should see if he's up at the memorial garden. My grandmother was buried there. Maybe he's visiting."

"I'll text Franco. He can check." Jake pulled Charlotte into a hug. He dropped a kiss on her temple. "It'll be okay."

What if he went near the water's edge? What if he slipped on the dock?

Charlotte's shaking increased. Jake grasped her arms and stepped back.

"Hey."

Charlotte scanned his black ski cap and heavy, gray sweater beneath a dark coat with dull, silver snaps. Blue jeans. Black boots.

Darks and lights of the lake.

What if Chuck had fallen? What if he was lying somewhere on the shoreline rocks?

Or worse.

What if?

"Charlotte. Charlotte, look at me." Jake tipped a finger under her chin. "Now."

She forced her gaze to trail up to his.

"What?"

"We will find him. Do you hear?" Jake snapped his fingers in front of her face. "You with me?"

"Yes? Yes."

"It'll be okay. Bea's making some calls. She'll get everyone out looking."

"Right." Charlotte shook herself, allowing her racing heartbeats to slow. He meant it, and she had to believe. She needed to get herself together.

"Thanks." She slowly pulled away. "Will you tell everyone where to go? I've got to start on the perimeter."

"Absolutely."

Charlotte wrapped a scarf around her neck, grabbed gloves, and headed for the door. "I'll call you."

"Good luck."

With Jake's words pushing her, Charlotte left the cottage and hurried toward the pavilion.

She blew into her gloves and pulled her jacket tighter. The temperature had dropped or the wind increased.

Or both.

She put the hood up and re-wrapped her scarf twice, adjusting the wool to cover her mouth.

Where are you, Dad?

On the dock she spied a lone couple walking hand-in-hand, despite the bitterness of the weather and the slick surface. There were those who walked Lakeside every day, 365 days a year, regardless of what Mother Nature threw at them. Her father had been one of those people, years ago. Where did his memory take him?

Skirting the boarded-up Hotel Lakeside, Charlotte hurried past the sailing club, the equally deserted basketball and volleyball courts, and the miniature golf course. Her head swiveled back and forth like a bobblehead doll—searching, searching.

She rounded the lakefront gazebo. Taking a sharp right, she left the path and walked beneath the trees toward the playground and the shuffleboard courts. Sweeping the park, she looped back around to the waterfront. A northern swath of fog obscured Kelleys Island, an unidentifiable mass in the distance.

Charlotte quickened her pace. Things could get worse before they got better. Additional snow would make the search more difficult.

She was running out of time.

She picked up the pace, and her heeled boots skidded beneath her. Catching herself on a nearby tree, Charlotte glanced again to the north. The cloud mass rolled toward land like a tumbleweed left to its own devices. Growing. Ominous.

"Chuck. Chuck!" Panic built in Charlotte's chest. "Dad, where are you?" Her voice grew raspy, and she hurried past a red farmhouse, a flat-roofed mid-century, and several multi-million-dollar Victorian mansions, all in the same row.

The wind whistled through the trees, a muffled off-key pitch. The shaking Charlotte had tamped down earlier began again. Splitting off from the path, she hung a right at the east gate booth, a smaller, less-impressive offspring of the large main entrance of the community. The gate gaped wide.

Please tell me he stayed inside the gates.

Charlotte's feet grew numb, her toes pinched in the impractical footwear. She faced the entrance. Like Chuck, she had a choice—keep to the Lakeside property or head toward Marblehead. Though it was less than a block to the village line, there were so many places he could get lost if he'd left the perimeter fence.

A crunch of tires on snow.

Charlotte turned, and a vehicle pulled beside her. Dana rolled down the driver's side window. In the back seat sat Trinity.

"Heard about Chuck," Dana said. "No sign of him, yet?"

Charlotte shook her head. "Nothing. I'm worried he might have gone outside the gates."

"I'll check Marblehead," Dana said. "We'll find him. It'll be okay, Charlotte. I just know it."

"It'll be okay. It'll be okay," Trinity parroted, her sing-song voice full of childish hope.

Charlotte's smile wobbled. "I wish I had her confidence."

"You want me to stop by the police station?" Dana said. "One of my in-laws is a cop."

"Thanks." Charlotte nodded. "We need all the help we can get."

"It'll be okay. It'll be okay, Miss Charlotte." Trinity waved a mittened hand, and the car pulled through and disappeared around the bend.

It may never be okay again.

But Charlotte needed it to be okay.

It *had* to be okay.

She wanted to tell her father she was sorry for ignoring his calls.

She wanted to tell him she was sorry for not giving him a chance.

But even if she found Chuck, she wasn't sure he'd really understand.

Please don't let it be too late.

Going with her gut, Charlotte headed south inside the fence line. At the corner of Poplar and 6th Street sat the entrance to the memorial garden, where her father had laid the ashes of his mother. Fresh tire tracks marred the snow-covered street. Franco must have already been there, but it wouldn't hurt to take a look for herself.

The memorial garden provided Lakesiders with a final resting place for the cremated remains of their loved ones, so their ashes could become one with the soil. Charlotte had not returned to Lakeside for the funeral of Grandma Anne Sutton, the donor of her middle name. She regretted that now.

Having no idea where her grandmother was buried, she took the most obvious route past a central pond and focused on the area at the rear of the park where pebbled nature trails wound in and out of the surrounding woods. The grounds crew, a staff of large proportions during season, scaled back to just a couple of year-round workers in the off-season. Dark, naked stalks, unpruned perennials left to their own devices, poked up through mounds of snow and ice.

Charlotte took a path to the right. Heart racing and her breath a puff of gray-white, she wound her way through the trees.

"Chuck. Dad, where are you?" Charlotte's yells came out hushed, as if Mother Nature had dampened the volume. Traveling the southern trails and finding no one, she turned onto the northern path.

On a dilapidated bench, tucked in a far corner of the park beneath a leaning tree with a huge knot in its side, Charlotte found Chuck. Slumped on a pile of snow-covered leaves, sticks, and other natural debris that had chosen the seat as an end-of-life resting place, he still wore his pajamas but had slipped boots on his feet and a hat on his head. His eyes were closed. His bare hands lay, palm up, in his lap.

"Dad?"

Chuck did not respond.

"Dad? Oh, God. Dad?" Charlotte stepped closer, her foot landing on a brittle stick.

Crack.

Chuck awoke. Hair poking out in all directions, coat buttons askew, and eyes wide with fear, he looked like a startled squirrel, unsure if he should run or wait to see if the human girl in front of him would pass on by.

A flush of heat rushed to Charlotte's heart, and her stomach heaved. She folded over and vomited into the bushes. And again. Gasping, she swiped her mouth.

"Oh, thank God."

Chuck's eyes dimmed. "Charlie?" He blinked. "Is that you?"

"Yeah, Dad." Charlotte dropped down on the bench beside him, barely aware of the cold of the snow or the crunch of the leaves she was crushing beneath her. Her gloved hand slipped around her father's cold one. "Oh! You're nearly frozen." She yanked off her gloves and rubbed her father's hands—like chilled leather—between her own, lifting them to her mouth and breathing warmth into his fingers. Her skin was smooth and pale, Chuck's chapped and red. Age spots branched up and over his knuckles.

She was swept back to when she was little. Her hands had been small then, fragile in her father's grasp. Now, she felt bigger, stronger.

Her father small. Fragile.

As if he had shrunk to nothing during his walk.

As if he would simply disappear like a pile of dust into the earth at their feet. Disappear like so many others before him.

"Where am I, exactly?" Chuck said.

"The memorial garden."

"I didn't know."

"I know, Dad."

"I didn't know where I was."

"It's okay."

Charlotte pressed her father's cold palms into her own shaking ones. They breathed in tandem. Chuck's head turned this way and that, taking in his location beneath the tree with the large knot in its side.

"I didn't know how to get home, Charlie."

"I'll text Jake and let him know where we are." Charlotte pulled out her phone. "He can bring up the car."

The chill and the wet of the bench filtered up through the leaves. Another shiver ran up her spine. Feeling her physical response, Chuck placed an arm around her shoulders and pulled her to him.

"You're shaking, kid."

"It's nothing."

Chuck patted her knee as if it were her, the daughter, who had gotten lost and he, the father, who had gone out looking, a worrying panic working its way through *his* system.

"At least I didn't go outside the gates."

"It's a good thing, Dad." Charlotte sucked in another deep, steadying breath. In. Out.

Chuck patted his daughter's knee again. "Thanks, kid."

"You're welcome." The chill seeped deeper into Charlotte's bones, into her soul. Her limbs felt leaden. The cold burrowed down to the core of who she thought she was, though she wasn't sure she could recognize herself anymore. Her body ached, the adrenaline from the search spent and useless to her now. She touched her temple. Her foggy brain couldn't quite catch up.

Is that what Alzheimer's feels like? A foggy brain?

"You're a right fine daughter, Charlie," Chuck said, "if I never told you. I probably didn't, but you're a right fine daughter."

Charlotte swallowed. What if she'd truly lost him? What kind of a daughter would she have been then?

"Thanks, Dad," she croaked.

"Hell of a writer, too."

"Thanks."

"I'm... I'm really, really proud of you, kid."

"Daddy?"

"Yes, Charlie."

Charlotte leaned into him. "That's all I ever wanted."

It was. Given a second chance, she wanted for her father to love her, be proud of her, and to see her for who she was.

A writer and his daughter.

His biggest fan.

"I'm proud of you, too," she said. "And I'm really sorry."

"Sorry? For what?"

"For not finding you sooner."

"It's all right. Wasn't *your* fault. It was mine." Chuck's fingers tightened around her shoulder. "Besides, we all have something to be sorry about. You found me quick enough."

"I think—"

"Yes, Charlie?"

"I think maybe we found each other." Charlotte squeezed her father's cold hand.

"Each other?"

"Yeah. It just took us some time. About 10 years."

Chuck let out a whoosh of white breath. His hand squeezed hers back. "It's the final inning that really matters."

Charlotte stood. A fat, wet snowflake hit her cheek. She glanced up at the sky. The cloud mass was practically upon them.

"Come on." She helped her father stand. "Let's go home."

Chuck smiled, his teeth a bright contrast to the drear of their surroundings.

"That sounds pretty good, Charlie. Real good."

"Yes, it does."

"I love you, kid."

"I love you, too, Dad."

36

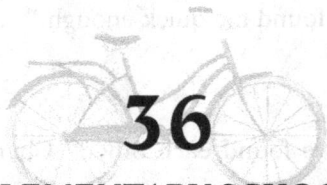

ELEMENTARY SCHOOL

Six-year-old Charlotte gripped the lip of the hull, her fingers wet with lake water. Waves slapped against the blue trim of her father's Sunfish, a boat with a striped sail of burnt orange and white.

"Let's start with the basics, kid," Daddy said. "When you're on a boat, left is?"

"Port." Charlotte giggled; she'd known that since she was three. "Right is starboard."

"Good show, Charlie. That's my girl."

With a flick of a wooden arm, the Sunfish took a sedate turn toward Kelleys Island.

"Here's the tiller. It steers Old Betty, see?"

Seagulls squawked above, and a dead fish floated by, the smell stinging the inside of Charlotte's nose. A swirl of icy water breached the side and crept over her fingertips. Bumps of cold dotted her arms.

The waves seemed higher at eye level than they did when Charlotte played on the strip of lawn between Sutton's Choice and the lake. Her eyes grew wide as the boat drifted past the L-dock. The lifejacket lay heavy on her shoulders, but she was glad of its warmth.

"I learned to sail on this boat, kid. Ol' Betty has been in our family a long, long time."

Her daddy adjusted a line.

"I'll teach you proper this summer, just like my daddy taught me."

"Fun," Charlotte whispered.

Sort of. She wasn't exactly sure yet.

The boat mimicked the motion of the waves beneath them. The lake looked so big—like they'd never return to land and would just float away together on a great adventure. Charlotte glanced back at the dock, now well behind them. There were no other boats on the water, but racks and racks sat by the shoreline in preparation for Memorial Day and the start of the season.

"It'll be a while before you're big enough to sail on your own, but I'll teach you the best I can," Daddy said, shifting the tiller. "We'll get you into lessons at the sailing center as soon as you're old enough. After a sailing test, you can go out on the lake by yourself."

"But I want to go with you, Daddy. Please? You'll take me, won't you?"

"Of course, I will."

Her father's aftershave briefly masked the dead fish odor. His arm extended behind Charlotte's shoulder, a bracing comfort. He pointed the boat toward a strip of land.

"All right, kid, what's that in the distance?"

"South Bass Island?"

"That's right, and straight ahead?"

Charlotte considered the distant lump of land. "Kelleys Island?"

"Yep, kid, two for two." Daddy motioned toward a tiny plot of trees. "See that? To your left? Port side? That's Mouse Island. Someday you'll even be a good enough sailor to take 'Ol Betty out for the race around it. The sailing club gives a trophy to the winner each year. I still have mine in a box somewhere. I won it when I was just a few years older than you are now."

"That sounds scary." Charlotte's stomach fluttered. She was pretty sure she didn't want to race. Pretty sure she'd lose.

"I don't wanna race, Daddy. It's too far."

"But you're in the big leagues now. Gotta swing for the fences. All right, then, coming about. Duck your head."

The metal pole swung above her—the attached sail flapping, taking on a life of its own. Charlotte ducked, and her father gave her a line. His big hand folded lightly over her tiny one.

"Hold this tight."

The sail went taunt and the boat cut through the water with sudden speed, hurtling them forward like a dolphin she'd seen in a movie once. The wind whipped through her hair, tossing it about her face in thick tangles. Charlotte's heart beat faster.

Oh.

She glanced up. Her father grinned at her.

"You're a natural, kid."

"Thanks, Daddy."

So fun. Charlotte liked sailing very much, even if she would never be very good at it. She reached out, sneaking her small hand again into her father's big one.

37

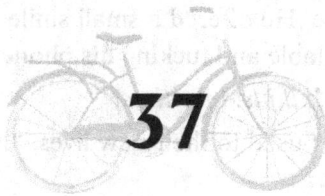

Charlotte pulled on a pair of tennis shoes and rummaged through her clothes for a warm jacket. She glanced at her phone. It was almost time.

She stood at the top of the steps and hollered to the house, at large. "You guys ready to go?"

Her father laughed, his response filtering up from the first floor.

"Just waiting on you, kid."

Charlotte hurried down the stairs. Chuck had donned a sweater and all-weather jacket and sat watching a Cleveland baseball game from his recliner.

"Can't wait to get out on the lake with you lot. Even if I have to miss the last two innings." There was a gleam in Chuck's eyes. "Worth it. Completely worth it."

Charlotte nodded. "I just hope we don't freeze. I can't believe there was still ice a couple of weeks ago."

"We won't freeze, Charlie. It's April Fool's Day. As the old saying goes, luck is what happens when preparation meets opportunity." Chuck patted his heavy coat. "I'm a fool, but I'm also prepared."

"Whatever you say, Dad."

Adam clomped down the stairs wearing a black hoodie, black windbreaker, black beanie, and black gloves.

Chuck snorted. "You getting ready to rob a bank, son?"

"What?"

"Nothing, kid. Very fashionable."

Adam's eyebrows shot up at his father's teasing, and he exchanged a look with Charlotte. He offered a small smile before grabbing his earphones from the table and tucking his phone in his pocket.

We'll be all right. It'll just take time.

They'd have to get used to their new lives. "Normal" came at an unusually high price.

"Let's roll," the teen said.

An awkward pack of mules, the three trailed each other down the waterfront path to the marina. Jake's boat, one of about a dozen in the water, bobbed at the furthest end of the pier. He had taken it out of storage at the first sign of spring.

Seagulls perched on the pylons of each slip, their screeching giving Charlotte chills and a warm feeling, all at the same time. Jake waved from where he stood waiting next to the *Erie Mermaid*. Sydney sat at attention beside him.

Charlotte tugged at her scarf, folding it against her ears, and a sudden gust of wind hit her. "Bea would say it's colder than a witch's ass out here."

Adam laughed. Leading the way, he strolled down the wooden planks. Chuck fell into step behind him. The seagulls, interrupted from their lookout, took flight in waves. Taking up the rear, Charlotte thought back to the many trips she'd enjoyed out on the water with her father when she was young. She'd learned everything about boating from him. Chuck had owned a motorboat, but Charlotte had preferred the sailboat.

She raised her voice above the squawking gulls. "Dad, do you still have Old Betty?"

"What?"

"The Sunfish. Do you still have the sailboat?"

Chuck smiled. "Ah. Old Betty. She was a fine ol' girl. She wasn't getting enough use, so I donated her to the sailing club a couple of years after you left. I sold the motorboat, too. I still see Old Betty on the water, from time to time, though. They've kept her in good shape."

"Do you know how to sail, Adam?" Charlotte said.

"Yeah. I took lessons."

"He's almost as good on the water as you are," Chuck said. "You two should go out this summer."

"Sure." Adam glanced over his shoulder. "I love to sail."

"Me, too." Charlotte smiled. "We could two-man it out and around Mouse Island, but damn well not today. The water looks positively frigid."

"A bit," Chuck said. "And I dare say the two of you aren't as small as you used to be. You'd be a tangle of arms and legs if you tried to tandem."

Charlotte grinned. "Fair. Well, then we could rent two boats and both enter the race this summer, just for fun."

Adam nodded. "I'm game."

As they approached Jake, Sydney bounded forward. She wrapped her body around Charlotte's legs and thrust her nose up under her hand.

Charlotte knelt down. "Hi, beautiful girl."

The dog bared teeth.

"The smile still freaks me out. Simply terrifying."

Jake laughed. "It's been months. You should be used to it by now. Obviously, she likes you as much as I do. Welcome aboard." He dropped a cool kiss on her lips and offered his hand.

A flood of warmth crept into her chilled fingers as he helped her climb into the boat. A glance at Jake, and she knew he felt it, too.

Their relationship had grown in leaps, and a future with him in it was a possibility that excited her.

"Winds are coming out of the west at just a couple of knots," Jake said. "I don't expect too much chop. Still going to be cold, but the sun's out, at least. Grab a seat under the bimini. It'll help block the wind."

Chuck and Charlotte did as instructed. Sydney jumped into the captain's chair, and Jake took the wheel. Dexterous as a cat, Adam climbed onto the bow, undid the bowline, and waited for the signal to toss it off.

"Everybody settled?" Jake said.

"Yep." Charlotte glanced at her father. He lounged back against the seat with his arms spread wide on the back of the cushions on either side. He'd stretched out his legs in front of him and crossed his ankles. A grin spread ear-to-ear.

Charlotte had loved Lake Erie forever, but Chuck had loved it for much, much longer. He'd grown up on the shores like she had; the water was his friend as much as it was hers. They had that in common.

"Let her rip, Jake." Chuck closed his eyes and dipped his chin to his chest.

Charlotte laughed. "Really? Spring has sprung. We're finally out on the lake, and you're going to take a nap?"

"Hell yes. There's nothing like the wind and water to make me sleepy."

Charlotte smiled.

"If this is the last boat ride I remember, Charlie, I'd like to make it count."

The smile dropped from Charlotte's lips. Would her father remember anything of this day in a week? A month? A year?

Or would the brief moment in time fade to nothing for him—just a whisper on the wind—a ghost of a memory he wouldn't hold onto while she and Adam did?

At war with no one but herself, Charlotte pulled her phone from her pocket and took a couple of pictures of the marina and shoreline. The boat turned toward open water.

"Come on back, Adam," Jake said. "We're clear."

The teen crawled to the edge of the deck, jumped down, and took a seat on the other side of Chuck. Pulling his headphones from his pocket, he put up his hood and settled in.

Brisk as it was, the views from the water would never grow old. The Lakeside pavilion and dock spread wide like welcoming arms—an inviting panorama. As quickly as the weather warmed up and the snow melted, the landscapers had raked and mulched the flower beds decorating the grounds. By Memorial Day, the community would be flush with early spring flowers. Dubbed "Ohio's most beautiful mile," in some past publicity effort, Lakeside had earned the term.

At least in Charlotte's eyes.

She couldn't wait to see her hometown in full spring bloom for the first time in a decade.

"There's a blanket in the cabin if you're cold," Jake said.

"Thanks. Good idea." Charlotte ducked through the door leading down below. The cabin was compact and functional, with a mattress beneath the aft, a tiny head, and a kitchenette. Blankets lay neatly stacked beneath a flat-screen TV.

"It's nice, Jake," Charlotte said, returning topside. She dropped a blanket in her father's lap. "You could live on your boat if you needed to."

"A bit cramped for me. An overnight on one of the islands is about all I can handle. I should take you up to Canada sometime this summer—a day trip to Pelee Island."

"I'd love that."

Charlotte held up a blanket and waved it at Adam. He shook his head, not bothering to take the earphones out of his ears. She sat down by her father and covered up.

"Sorry. Colder than I expected," Jake said. "We'll just head east toward the lighthouse and loop around."

"You're in charge, son." Chuck did not lift his chin from his chest. "Any time spent on the water is time well spent."

Moments later, they passed the quarry, where limestone in the area was processed. Jake dipped in closer to shore, skirting the barge and the wake of a ferry puttering north.

Charlotte pulled a piece of gum from her pocket. The crinkle of paper prompted Sydney to hop down from the captain's chair and take a spot beside her. The dog pressed her body tightly against Charlotte's side, lifting a paw and placing it on her arm.

"No gum for you, girl."

"She's a terrible beggar," Jake said. "Tell her to get down if it bothers you."

"Oh, it's no bother. She's warmer than the blanket." Charlotte held out her phone, put her arm around the dog, and pressed her face against its fur. "Sydney, picture time." Turning, she leaned into her father. "What do you say, Dad? Selfie?"

Chuck's eyes popped open. "Selfie?"

Charlotte's cheek brushed stubble. "Come on. Smile."

"Whatever makes you happy, Charlie."

Charlotte adjusted the screen and took several shots. With chilled fingers, she zoomed in on one of the pictures.

"Oh, my gosh."

She held the phone out for her father to see.

Chuck stared down at the picture of the two of them.

Their matching, wavy hair—Charlotte's dark as a raven's feather, Chuck's sprinkled with gray.

Their deep brown eyes with flecks of yellow around the irises.

Their cupid lips—Charlotte's just a bit fuller than her father's.

"Twins. That's a fine picture, Charlie. A fine picture." Chuck swiped at a smear of moisture on his cheek. "Damned wind makes my eyes water."

"Let me see." Adam pulled his headphones from his ears and motioned to Charlotte's phone.

She handed it to him. Adam's eyes soaked in the picture, a frown playing at his lips.

"That's nuts."

"Let me take one of all three of you," Jake said.

"Come on, Adam," Charlotte said. "A family portrait."

"Nah." Adam shrugged and handed back the phone.

"Please," Chuck whispered.

Adam glanced at Charlotte.

She nodded. "Please."

Adam shrugged again and leaned closer. Jake snapped a photo.

Charlotte retrieved her phone. "Triplets." Adam's skin was a shade or two darker than hers, she assumed thanks to his mother's heritage, but otherwise there truly was no doubting the Sutton gene.

"Thanks, kids." Chuck patted each of his children's knees.

"Sure. Whatever." Adam stood and headed to the back of the boat. Plunking down on the rear cushions, he stuffed his headphones back into his ears and yanked the hoodie up.

Jake mouthed "Sorry."

"It's fine." Charlotte would have responded the same at Adam's age.

"I suppose it'll take some adjusting," Jake said.

"I know."

"What will?" Chuck asked, a hint of confusion in his voice.

"My decision, Dad," Charlotte said. "To move back to Sutton's Choice."

"Ah, yes. Give him time. He'll grow used to it, Charlie."

Charlotte nodded. It was true. She and Adam would rely on each other to get through the rough times that were coming, but together they'd also enjoy what they both wanted most—time spent with their mutual father.

Maybe, someday, we'll even be friends.

"How's it going with the move," Jake said. "Are you mostly packed up?"

"Yep. I'm heading back to Pittsburgh tomorrow to pick up the rest of my things and put Mom's condo on the market. I'll come back right after the Saturday kick-off open house for Designer Greens."

"Sounds like you're going to be really busy," Jake said.

Charlotte laughed. "But it's good busy. I'm just so glad Tania agreed to let me go fully remote."

Jake grinned. "We all are."

"Right." Chuck closed his eyes. "Finally, my daughter has returned to the nest."

"Anything new from Grant about your idea to expand the newspaper to include a Beyond Business advertising agency?" Jake said.

"Still discussing it. He set up an appointment with Tania for next month. I think it could happen. She seems interested in franchising."

"That's fantastic."

"Proud of you, kid." Chuck's eyes were still closed. His lips spread wide in a smile, and he tilted his chin into the wind. "Thanks for bringing us out, Jake. This is great. Just great. Didn't think I'd get the chance again."

"Anytime."

The boat passed an 1800s limestone house built by one of the earliest settlers to the area long before it became a bed and breakfast. They curved further around the mainland, and, suddenly, the Marblehead Lighthouse popped into view. The white beacon fronted a rocky shore and clumps of trees.

"She's always so beautiful from the water," Charlotte said.

"Agreed." Jake crept along and eventually turned north toward Kelleys Island. Charlotte soaked in the sights, knowing it would not be the last time she'd get the experience. Island cottages fronted the shore, clinging to the edge like sandcastles bracing for a wave. The details of the buildings were thrown into stark relief against the foreground of deep gray lake water. The weak sun slipped behind a cloud and popped back out again.

Charlotte looked back at Adam, slouched on the seat at the aft of the boat. He lounged in a corner, his eyes closed. His head nodded with a rhythm only he could hear, and his fingers tapped the beat on his knee. Adam opened his eyes, catching Charlotte in mid-look. He jutted his chin skyward, and she smiled. Adam returned a faint smile of his own. He closed his eyes again and resumed tapping. In that moment, he was more kin to Chuck than Charlotte was.

She studied father and son—worshipping the sun, the wind, and water.

We'll be all right.

She let the cool air fill her lungs and snuggled closer to her father under the blanket.

"What a fine day," Chuck mumbled, grasping his daughter's hand beneath the blanket. "I'm so glad you came home. Love you, kid."

"I love you, too, Dad."

"You're going to be a fantastic editor. My first-round pick. No doubt about it."

"Thanks. Zara's a big help, but I'll try my best."

"Zara?"

Charlotte nodded. "The retired editor from Cleveland?"

"Oh. Right." Chuck squeezed her hand. "It'll all be fine. You'll be more than fine."

"Thanks, Dad."

A half an hour later, they'd skirted the waterfront and circled around toward home. Chuck had succumbed to sleep, his lips turned up slightly at the corners.

"Can we swing past the Lakeside dock one more time, before we head in," Charlotte whispered. "I don't want to wake him, just yet."

"Of course." Jake turned the boat.

If she could make a wish, it would be that the Suttons would only ever have pleasant memories, from then on, of time spent together on the water, their common love of the lake something Alzheimer's could never erase.

She was glad to finally be home.

Charlotte spotted a glimpse of the little cottage next to the hotel.

She'd made the right choice.

Sutton's Choice.

38

10 YEARS LATER

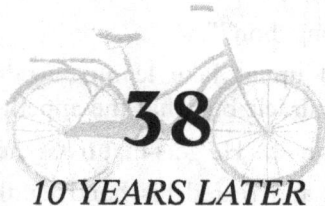

Her daughter's laughter drifted on the lakefront breeze over the waves and back to Charlotte sitting in the rocker on the porch of Sutton's Choice. Like a masthead on a schooner, Isabella perched on the bow of Adam's sailboat as he skimmed along the shoreline. Her tanned face tilted into the wind, and her black hair streamed out behind her. At six, Charlotte's daughter was as small and fierce and happy as Sammy and looked more and more like him every day, too. Mama Macon nearly popped with pride. There were hints of Chuck and Charlotte in her, of course, but Sammy's Latino genes were winning the battle. Though Charlotte's own hair had tested her patience all through childhood, Isabella's grew more lush and curlier every day. Tired of dealing with the tangles, Charlotte had begged Sammy to give their daughter a pixie cut like her own, but Isabella had insisted she'd have none of that.

Absolutely not.

Isabella's wild hair, curls and all, was hers and hers alone.

Charlotte's foot set her favorite rocker *thwap, thwap, thwapping*— wood against weathered wood. The baby in her arms started to fuss, and the young Australian shepherd napping at her feet immediately stood at alert, her nose resting on Charlotte's knee. One blue eye and one brown gazed up at her.

Charlotte patted the dog. "It's okay, Betty girl. I'm not hurting him." She plucked the bottle from her son's mouth and adjusted a towel over her shoulder. Lifting the baby, she set his blonde, downy head to nuzzle against her cheek. Shuddering, he burped loudly in her ear.

"Good one, buddy."

"You need anything, hon?"

Charlotte looked up at Jake leaning against the doorframe. "Nope. Charlie the miracle baby has the appetite of a horse."

Her husband laughed. "He gets that from me."

Jake strode over and rested his hand lightly on his son's tiny back. His lips touched the top of her head before he leaned down to kiss Charlie.

Charlotte smiled, and the rocker continued thwapping.

"Long road to get to here but worth it," she said. "Genetics are a funny thing. I suppose we're going to have to talk to Sammy soon about how to explain our family to our children, huh?"

"That's an understatement," Jake said. "We'll figure it out."

Nine years since their marriage. Eight since Jake was told he'd likely never be able to produce children. They'd been grateful to Sammy when he'd offered to do exactly what he'd joked about for years and made, in his words, a "Chammy deposit"—Isabella the result.

So different from Charlotte's own upbringing, Isabella's childhood had, so far, been filled with more fatherly love than one could ever ask for. Isabella called Jake "Daddy," but Sammy spent many hours every week with his daughter and the Sutton clan. Mama Macon served as a willing, joyful babysitter—on call 24-7. Sutton's Choice included a veritable revolving door for fathers and family and friends... and friends that were family and fathers.

They'd been told Isabella would be their only child. Then, against all odds, the Sutton family tree continued its half-sibling ways, its limbs branching to include Charlie, their sweet little biological surprise. He'd arrived a month premature and spent some time in the NICU before finally being allowed to come home.

The new generation of Sutton half-siblings would raise eyebrows and questions. In appearance, Isabella was her little brother's opposite. Charlie looked like he might keep Jake's white-blonde hair and Charlotte's pale skin.

"Could you whistle for them to come in?" Charlotte said. "Isabella needs a shower before the memorial service. Mama is saving us a seat, but the place will be packed."

"Sure, hon." Jake left the porch, the Aussie following at a close heel.

* * * * *

Charlotte handed Charlie to Adam and bent down to her daughter's level.

"Remember, kid, we'll need to be very quiet during the service."

"I know, Mom." Isabella groaned, rolling her eyes. "You told me. Come on, Sam-I-Am. Let's go sit."

"She's got this, Char," Sammy said.

"Come onnnn, Sam-I-Am." Isabella tugged Sammy's hand.

Though Charlotte didn't usually like nicknames, Isabella's choice for Sammy had tickled the hairdresser and was a perfect fit. He'd been reading Dr. Seuss to his child from the day of her birth.

Sammy allowed his little dynamo to lead him away, and Adam trailed after with Baby Charlie. Isabella skipped through the entrance to the memorial garden and toward Mama Macon, sitting in the third row of chairs. Beside her sat Mrs. T and her Chihuahua, Snuggles II, who sported a yellow daisy tied to its collar. At the other end of the row sat the Warren family and Dana and Jimmy Stanner with their youngest daughter, Demi.

"Saved you a seat, Bella," Demi said, giggling and patting the chair beside her. Isabella ran ahead down the aisle.

Charlotte felt a tap on her shoulder.

295

"Glad to see you lot."

She turned and was folded into Franco Bellimer's arms.

"Of course, Mr. B. You know how sorry we are."

Jake shook the man's hand. "Bea was one of a kind."

"We had some great years together before the cancer took her," Bellimer said. "Good times in spades for a couple of faded, washed-up old farts like us. That's more than I can say of a lot of married couples."

"True," Charlotte said.

"If it weren't for your father, it might never have been," Bellimer said. "All those hours sitting in the memory care unit in his last couple of years, just the three of us watching sports. That's when Bea finally loosened up. Stubborn as the day is long, that woman. Took me years to wear her down enough to go on a proper date."

Charlotte laughed. "That's because you weren't any good at those effing darts."

"Damned right. I was always worried if I ever really pissed her off, she could have killed me with one of those things. Deadly aim."

"She's up there in heaven throwin' darts with Chuck, now, I'd imagine," Jake said.

Bellimer nodded. "He's introduced the old girl around to everyone and given her a proper welcome, to be sure."

"I bet." Charlotte smiled. "Dad had a way of making people feel at ease."

"He sure did." Bellimer rubbed his bald head. His usual tweed jacket hung looser than normal, and Charlotte was worried about him. He intended to leave the paper for good and move down to Florida by himself to a retirement community in the fall. She couldn't imagine running the paper without him, but at least they'd have the rest of the summer to train Adam as his replacement.

Her brother would be the perfect reporter to fill the little man's shoes. After graduating college and spending a year in Europe, traveling all over and writing about his experiences, Adam had not landed in a big city, as she'd done two decades before. Instead, he'd returned to Lakeside. It was where he belonged, he'd told her.

They were family, and family was home.

Home.

"Bea's service is starting in about 10 minutes," Bellimer said. "I've got to make the rounds. Don't forget to join me for a toast at the bar after."

"Of course," Charlotte said.

Franco Bellimer nodded, patted Charlotte on the shoulder, and shuffled off.

"Shall we take a seat?" Jake said.

"You go ahead without me. I'll be just a minute."

Jake bent down and kissed Charlotte's cheek. "Take your time, hon."

*   *   *   *   *

Skirting the pavilion, she slipped down the memorial garden path to where she'd found her father—lost—that fateful, snowy day. Sinking onto a new bench she and Adam had donated to Lakeside, Charlotte leaned back and looked up at the branches. The leaves were in full bloom, providing a shade her father would appreciate.

"Hey. It's me." Charlotte shifted, getting comfortable. "Bea's going to have a beautiful day for the funeral. There's a dart tournament and reception at the bar after. Drinks on the house, of course."

She took a breath.

"Charlie's growing like a weed, Dad. His legs are getting so long. I think he's going to be tall like you and me. Did I tell you Bella starts school soon? The summer has gone by so fast this year. Crazy."

Charlotte patted the arm of the bench, smooth metal beneath her palm. "Anyway, I just wanted to stop by and say 'hi'."

She closed her eyes, thinking back to the several years Chuck had lived after her return. His final months had been difficult. He hadn't recognized her near the end. Alzheimer's had taken those memories from him. It had been hardest for Adam, though. Chuck had lost memories of his younger child much, much sooner.

They'd spent hours and hours reading to their father, either their own writings or old newspaper stories or entries from his many journals, an entire box of which they'd found tucked away in the attic. The time spent together, just the three of them, had helped Chuck relive his past and had allowed the Sutton siblings to finally get to really *know* him.

And to say goodbye.

Despite all odds, Chuck had been the glue that held the family together.

Charlotte sighed. She was grateful for that.

Maybe, someday, little Charlie would learn to sail, and Isabella would marry at the hotel where her parents and grandparents had wed. Maybe, Adam would take over the running of the paper and the advertising agency.

Someday.

Like her father, Charlotte would eventually say goodbye to all the people she had chosen to love in the ridiculous, beautiful, quaint little waterfront town of Lakeside, Ohio.

It wasn't really a choice. Someday would come.

Turning, Charlotte ran her fingers over the memorial plaque at her back.

In loving memory of Charles Adam Sutton—You're in the big leagues now, kid.

A slight breeze lifted the short hairs on her neck. She glanced up again, seeking the sliver of blue sky between the branches.

"I miss you, too, Dad. Wish you were here."

A Note from the Author

Thank you, readers, for spending time in my fictional world.

I had three goals in writing this story. I wanted to connect with those who experienced childhood trauma and/or complicated family relationships. I wanted to set my story in the quaintest of waterfront towns (the very real Lakeside, Ohio). And I wanted to spark conversations about dementia and, in particular, Alzheimer's disease. I've seen so many loved ones impacted by Alzheimer's, either as patients or caregivers. In *Finding Sutton's Choice*, I allowed this horrible illness to do something rare… to bring a fractured family closer in a positive, healing way.

For those of you lucky enough to personally know Lakeside, Ohio, I've sprinkled our real town with a bit of fictional fairy dust. No such street as Pine exists. No such cottage named Sutton's Choice exists. No bar is currently attached to the marina that sits just beyond the gates. Regardless of the liberties I've taken, for the sake of the story, I hope my wild imagination still captures the essence of Lakeside. She is a wonderfully unique little town… one I am very blessed to call home.

Finding Sutton's Choice came to life thanks to the support of many friends and family members. In particular, I couldn't have done this without you, Mike, my husband and first and last reader (always). Your confidence in me surpasses my own.

Pam McCarthy, writing cheerleader and English teacher extraordinaire, thank you for offering your own personal stories and an editorial eye. Jill Collins, you were one tough grammarian, but your lessons, decades ago, have served me well.

Susan Poole, you arrived in my life right on time with your killer red pen, sympathetic commiseration, and all the feels as we shared similar debut author journeys.

Editor-in-Chief Michael T. Braun, editor Michelle Murray, and the entire staff at Orange Hat Publishing/Ten16 Press, I am grateful for your attention to detail, limitless patience, and unwavering commitment to taking a chance on me and my story. Dana Breunig, you deserve a special shout-out for an outstanding, Rusty-Banana-infused cover. Oh, my heart.

Last but certainly not least, a huge "thank you" to my dozens of early readers—Mom, Elaine, friends and family members, critique group writers, Lakesiders, attorneys, medical professionals, and caregivers. You offered moral support, professional knowledge, and honest feedback before this book was remotely ready for mass consumption. I am overwhelmed with gratitude. Your input helped me improve my writing and elevate *Finding Sutton's Choice* to a place on a bookshelf.

Thank you all.

We did it. Together.

For book club discussion materials, speaker information, or to sign up for Brenda's newsletter, visit www.brendahaas.com.

www.ingramcontent.com/pod-product-compliance
Lightning Source LLC
Chambersburg PA
CBHW011220290326
41931CB00044B/3461